Congenital Müllerian Anomalies

Samantha M. Pfeifer

Editor

Congenital Müllerian Anomalies

Diagnosis and Management

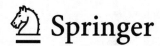 Springer

Editor
Samantha M. Pfeifer
Weill Cornell Medical College
New York, NY, USA

ISBN 978-3-319-80096-7   ISBN 978-3-319-27231-3   (eBook)
DOI 10.1007/978-3-319-27231-3

Printed on acid-free paper

This Springer imprint is published by Springer Nature
The registered company is Springer International Publishing AG Switzerland

Preface

Müllerian anomalies are rare conditions of female reproductive organ development. These anomalies may be asymptomatic or can present with delayed menarche, abdominal pain, or severe dysmenorrhea during puberty and adolescence, or even later in life with reproductive issues. As these anomalies are rare, they are often not considered in the differential diagnosis at the time of presentation, leading to a delay in diagnosis with subsequent risk of pain, loss of reproductive organs, and adverse effect on future fertility. In addition to the physical issues that can occur, these anomalies may have significant psychological implications as reproductive and sexual function may be affected. With the development of better imaging modalities, minimally invasive and innovative surgical techniques, and assisted reproductive technologies, there are now many more options for diagnosing and managing these anomalies and their impact on reproductive function.

Congenital Müllerian Anomalies: Diagnosis and Management is a comprehensive book intended to illustrate the current tools required to diagnose and treat these often complex conditions affecting reproductive function and fertility. It is ideally suited for the practicing gynecologist, reproductive endocrinologist, pediatrician, adolescent medicine specialist as well as allied health professionals, residents, fellows, and students interested in the topic. Chapter topics were chosen to cover all Müllerian anomalies, including those diagnosed during puberty and adolescence as well as anomalies typically presenting in later reproductive years. The anomalies are grouped into those resulting from vertical defects of development or lateral defects. Each chapter reviews the etiology, presentation and diagnosis, surgical and nonsurgical management options as well as discussing implications for fertility and treatment options. Chapter authors were selected by the editor for their expertise in the field. This book provides an up-to-date framework for understanding the presentation, diagnosis, and surgical and nonsurgical treatment options of Müllerian anomalies, with a focus on identifying and managing their impact on reproductive function and future fertility.

Weill Cornell Medical College
New York, NY

Samantha M. Pfeifer

Contents

The original version of this book was revised. An erratum to this book can be found at
DOI 10.1007/978-3-319-27231-3_13

Contributors

Veronica I. Alaniz, MD, MPH Department of Obstetrics and Gynecology, University of Michigan Health System, SPC , Ann Arbor, MI, USA

Heather Appelbaum, MD Division of Pediatric and Adolescent Gynecology, Cohen Children's Medical Center of NY/Northwell Medical Center, Hofstra North Shore LIJ School of Medicine, New Hyde Park, NY, USA

Marjan Attaran, MD Cleveland Clinic, Cleveland, OH, USA

Jeanne Choi-Rosen, MD Pediatric Radiology, Cohen Children's Medical Center of NY/Northwell Medical Center, Hofstra North Shore LIJ School of Medicine, New Hyde Park, NY, USA

M. Alexa Clapp, MD Obstetrics and Gynecology & Women's Health, Montefiore Medical Center, Albert Einstein College of Medicine, Bronx, NY, USA

Jennifer E. Dietrich, MD, MSc Obstetrics and Gynecology and Pediatrics, Texas Children's Hospital, Houston, TX, USA

Julie Hakim, MD Department of Obstetrics and Gynecology, Division of Pediatric Adolescent Gynecology, Baylor College of Medicine, Houston, TX, USA

S. Paige Hertweck, MD Kosair Children's Hospital, Louisville, KY, USA

Sari Kives, MD The Hospital for Sick Children, Pediatric Gynecology, Toronto, ON, Canada

Jovana Lekovich, MD Ronald O. Perelman and Claudia Cohen Center for Reproductive Medicine, New York, NY, USA

Erica B. Mahany, MD L4510 Women's Hospital, Ann Arbor, MI, USA

Kate McCracken, MD Kosair Children's Hospital Louisville, KY, USA

Nigel Pereira, MD Weill Cornell Medicine, New York, NY, USA

Kathryn Peticca, MD University of Pittsburgh School of Medicine, Magee-Womens Hospital, Pittsburgh, PA, USA

Samantha M. Pfeifer, MD Weill Cornell Medical College, New York, NY, USA

Staci E. Pollack, MD Obstetrics and Gynecology & Women's Health, Division of Reproductive Endocrinology & Infertility, Montefiore Medical Center, Albert Einstein College of Medicine, Bronx, NY, USA

Elisabeth H. Quint, MD Department of Obstetrics and Gynecology, University of Michigan Health System, SPC, Ann Arbor, MI, USA

Beth W. Rackow, MD Department of Obstetrics and Gynecology, Columbia University Medical Center, New York, NY, USA

Joseph S. Sanfilippo, MD, MBA University of Pittsburgh School of Medicine, Magee-Womens Hospital, Pittsburgh, PA, USA

Yolanda R. Smith, MD, MS L4510 Women's Hospital, Ann Arbor, MI, USA

Jamie Stanhiser, MD Cleveland Clinic, Cleveland, OH, USA

Shawna Tonick, MD Department of Obstetrics and Gynecology, Cohen Children's Medical Center of NY/Northwell Medical Center, Hofstra North Shore LIJ School of Medicine, New Hyde Park, NY, USA

Lauren Zakarin, MD Center for Women's Reproductive Care, New York, NY, USA

Part I

Etiology and Diagnosis

Müllerian Anomaly Classification Systems

Sari Kives

While genital malformations are relatively common, over the last 50 years there has yet to be a single classification system developed which is easily utilized and interpreted. There remains a need for a correct and clear method of categorization which will effectively guide therapeutic management.

The first attempt to classify female congenital anomalies goes back to the 1800s and lacks significant organization and clarity. Later in 1907, Strassman et al. first described these anomalies as either symmetric double malformations (didelphys, bicornuate, or septate) or asymmetric ones (unicornuate, with or without a rudimentary horn) [1].

The Jones and Rock Classification in 1953 [2] included defects of both midline fusion (e.g., bicornuate uterus), unilateral malformation and defects of canalization (e.g., transverse vaginal septum). This classification incorporated mullerian anomalies as well as complex malformations including vertical fusion defects (Fig. 1.1).

In 1979, Buttram and Gibbons developed the first widely accepted classification system based on their results from an analysis of 144 cases [3]. In this study, 44 patients had been exposed to DES and had an abnormal hysterosalpingogram and the remainder were patients discharged from hospital with a diagnosis of uterine anomaly. These anomalies were divided into five different groups based on the degree of failure of normal uterine anatomical development. The anomalies were also classified according to similar clinical presentations and pregnancy outcomes.

According to Buttram et al., class one (segmental mullerian agenesis/hypoplasia) most frequently presented with vaginal agenesis and was often associated with primary amenorrhea. Class two (unicornuate) most frequently presented with an abnormal shaped uterus and was associated with an increased incidence of preterm labor and abnormal presentation [4]. Class three (didelphys) most frequently presented with abnormal ultrasound findings and was also associated with preterm delivery [5]. Class four (bicornuate uterus) most frequently presented as an abnormally shaped uterus and also associated with premature labor, breach presentation, and cesarean delivery [4]. Finally, class five (septate uterus) was often incidentally discovered, but associated with a very high first trimester loss rate [3]. An additional category was included to take into account patients exposed to DES and having unique anomalies related to in utero exposure.

The first revision of this classification was in 1988 by the American Fertility Society (AFS), which was renamed the American Society for Reproductive medicine (ASRM) in 1995 [6]. The ASRM system is currently the most broadly used

S. Kives, M.D. (✉)
The Hospital for Sick Children, Pediatric
Gynecology, 555 University Avenue, Toronto, ON,
Canada, M1E 2L6
e-mail: kivess@smh.ca

© Springer International Publishing Switzerland 2016
S.M. Pfeifer (ed.), *Congenital Müllerian Anomalies*, DOI 10.1007/978-3-319-27231-3_1

The Jones Classification system

CHART 2. ETIOLOGICAL BASIS OF ANOMALY

	TYPE 1. DEFECT OF FUNDUS (With single cervix & vagina)
	A. Septate Uterus:
	Complete septum with non-communicating cavities.
	Partial septum with communicating cavities.
	B. Bicornuate Uterus.
	TYPE 2. DEFECT OF CERVIX AND/OR VAGINA (Single fundus)
Defect of Midline Fusion	A. Septate vagina, with single cervix.
	B. Single or septate vagina, with septate cervix.
	C. Single or septate vagina, with double cervix.
	D. Double vagina, with double cervix.
	TYPE 3. FAILURE OF FUSION AT ALL LEVELS.
	A. Double uterus, double cervix, double vagina.
	(Classical "uterus didelphys")
	MATURATION OF SINGLE MULLERIAN SYSTEM
Unilateral Maturation	A. Unilateral development, with absence of opposite tract.
	Unilateral maturation, with rudimentary opposite tract,
	which may or may not communicate with the functioning side
	DEFECT OF LONGITUDINAL CANALIZATION OF VAGINA.
Defect of Canalization	A. Transverse vaginal shelves or septa.
	B. Complete atresia of the vagina is the extreme degree of this type.

Jones W. Congenital Malformations Trans New Eng J Obs Gyn 1953 p. 83

Fig. 1.1 The Jones classification system. *Jones W. Congenital Malformations Trans New Eng J Obs Gyn 1953 p. 83*

system and contains seven basic groups based on the embryology of the mullerian system. The anomalies were organized according to the major uterine anatomic types, specifically the presence of each segment of the female reproductive tract, the outer contour of the uterine fundus, and the presence of a septum [6]. Vaginal anomalies are not a part of this classification system. However, the ASRM classification system allowed the user to indicate the uterine malformation type but in addition describe the associated variations of the vagina, cervix, tubes, ovaries, and urologic system [6]

An additional category for arcuate uterus was added to Buttram's original classification.

The ASRM classification system is based mainly on uterine malformations, which make up the vast majority of cases, making utilization of this classification easier. The classification, however, is rather subjective as it relies on pictures depicting these anomalies without any clear descriptive definitions. In response to this subjective diagnostic criteria, several authors have proposed supplementing the ASRM classification with additional morphometric criteria [7–9]

These proposed criteria specify the size of endometrial and fundal indentations to standardize the definition of septate and bicornuate anomalies.

The ASRM classification system remains widely accepted today. Limitations to the ASRM method include the lack of classification of congenital utero-vaginal anomalies and complex genitourinary anomalies (Fig. 1.2).

In 2004, Acien et al. [10] proposed a classification of congenital female malformations using the embryological–clinical classification and updated this system in 2011 [11]. The authors felt that all previous classifications systems were based solely on mullerian embryologic classifications and did not sufficiently explain, detect, or help treat the full spectrum of female genitourinary malformations. This new classification system incorporated the embryology as well as the pathogenesis of genital malformations 11 [8].

As per Acien et al., there were five possible locations for the origin of the six groups of malformations: (1) Agenesis or hypoplasia of the entire urogenital ridge, (2) Mesonephric anomalies with an absence of the Wolffian duct opening into the urogenital sinus and of the ureteral bud sprouting, (3) Isolated mullerian anomalies (similar to ASRM system), (4) Gubernaculum dysfunction, (5) Anomalies of the urogenital sinus, and (6) Malformative combinations.

This method allowed for classification of the full spectrum of genital malformations. The authors felt that, although a clinico-embryologic classification may be more complicated, it would allow for correct cataloguing as well as proper therapeutic planning for surgical correction of these anomalies. Prior classification systems were essentially based solely on lateral fusion defects of the mullerian ducts. Up-to-date embryological knowledge suggested that the mesonephric ducts and gubernaculum also played a role in the adequate development of the mullerian ducts and therefore should be included as part of the classification system [10].

While this method is comprehensive, it is not easily interpreted or utilized without the use of complex reference tables (Fig. 1.3).

In 2005, Oppelt et al. proposed a very detailed classification based on the Tumor Nodes Metastases (TMN) principles in oncology and labeled it as VCAUM (vagina, cervix, uterus, adnexa, and associated malformations) [12]. This was put forward as a response to prior classifications, which the authors noted were primarily limited to the uterus and vagina and disregarded malformations of the adnexa. Associated anomalies were also not incorporated into the previous classification systems. The aim of utilizing the TMN principles was to provide a description of the malformation that was individualized and as accurate and precise as possible [12]. This classification system allowed the assessment of the complete genital malformation which was not feasible with uterine-specific classification systems [12] (Fig. 1.4).

This classification is relatively straightforward to apply, however not easily interpreted or utilized without the use of appropriate tables.

In 2012, Grimibiz et al. developed a new approach to the classification incorporating both features of the ASRM model and Acien's embryological one [13]. This system was created by the European Society of Human Reproduction and Embryology and European Society for Gynecological Endoscopy (ESHRE-ESGE), under the working group CONUTA (CONgenital UTerine Anomalies). The goal was to replace previous classification systems, which were thought to be limited in the effective categorization of the anomalies, clinical usefulness, simplicity, and user-friendliness [13].

The final results of the working group was development of a classification system with the following characterisitics: (1) Anatomy is the basis for systematic categorization, (2) Deviation of uterine anatomy deriving from the same embryological area are the basis for design of the main classes, (3) Subclasses are anatomical variations of the main classes, and (4) Cervical and vaginal anomalies are classified as independent supplementary subclasses. Uterine anatomy remained the basis for the new system similar to other classification systems, but embryological origin was also adopted in the design of the main classes (Fig. 1.5).

TABLE 5
THE AMERICAN FERTILITY SOCIETY CLASSIFICATION OF MULLERIAN ANOMALIES

Patient's Name _____ Date _____ Chart # _____

Age _____ G _____ P _____ Sp Ab _____ VTP _____ Ectopic _____ Infertile Yes _____ No _____

Other Significant History (i.e. surgery, infection, etc.) _____

_____

HSG _____ Sonography _____ Photography _____ Laparoscopy _____ Laparotomy _____

EXAMPLES

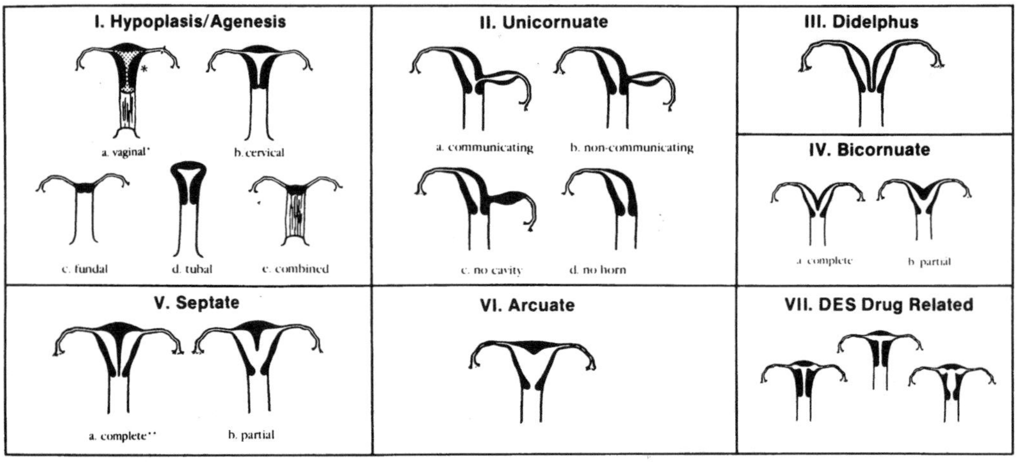

I. Hypoplasis/Agenesis	II. Unicornuate	III. Didelphus
a. vaginal* b. cervical c. fundal d. tubal e. combined	a. communicating b. non-communicating c. no cavity d. no horn	**IV. Bicornuate** a. complete b. partial

V. Septate	VI. Arcuate	VII. DES Drug Related
a. complete** b. partial		

* Uterus may be normal or take a variety of abnormal forms.
** May have two distinct cervices

Type of Anomaly

Class I	_____	Class V	_____
Class II	_____	Class VI	_____
Class III	_____	Class VII	_____
Class IV	_____		

Treatment (Surgical Procedures): _____

_____

_____

Prognosis for Conception & Subsequent Viable Infant*

_____ Excellent (> 75%)

_____ Good (50-75%)

_____ Fair (25%-50%)

_____ Poor (< 25%)

*Based upon physician's judgment.

Recommended Followup Treatment: _____

_____

_____

Property of
The American Fertility Society

Additional Findings: _____

_____

_____

Vagina: _____
Cervix: _____

Tubes: Right _____ Left _____
Kidneys: Right _____ Left _____

DRAWING

L   R

For additional supply write to:
The American Fertility Society
2140 11th Avenue, South
Suite 200
Birmingham, Alabama 35205

Fig. 1.2 AFS/ASRM classification of mullerian anomalies

Table II Illustrated relationship and classification of the pathogenic findings and anatomical figures with symptoms and pathology name, following an updated embryological and clinical classification of female genital tract malformations.

Aetiopathogenic anomaly	Anatomical findings	Pathology name	Clinical symptoms
1. Unilateral genito-urinary agenesis or hypoplasia			
1.1 With contralateral müllerian agenesis	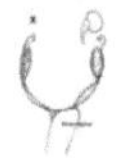	Rokitansky syndrome with URA	Primary amenorrhoea
1.2 Without contralateral agenesis	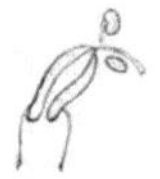	Unicornuate uterus with contralateral RA	No symptoms. Reproductive Breech present
2. Uterine duplicity with a blind hemivagina (or atresia) and ipsilateral RA, showing			
2.1 Large hematocolpos, blind hemivagina	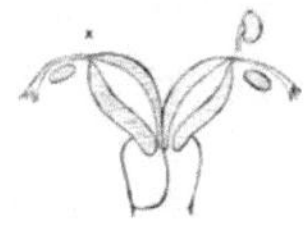	Didelphys or bicornuate uterus with blind hemivagina and ipsilateral RA	Pain. Intra and postmenstrual dysmenorrhoea Pelvic tumour Postmenstrual spotting
2.2 Like Gartner's pseudocyst	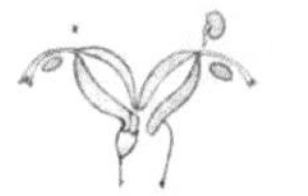	Bicornuate communicating uterus, athretic blind hemivagina and ipsilateral RA. Herlyn-Werner syndrome	Pain? Cyst in anterolateral wall of vagina. Postmenstrual spotting or vaginal discharge.
2.3 Partial reabsorption of the vaginal septum	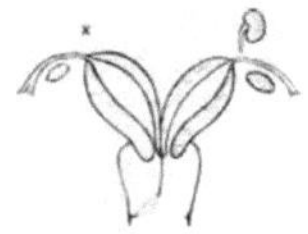	Didelphys or bicornis-bicollis uterus with a short septum or buttonhole, and URA	No symptoms. Dyspareunia. Reproductive. Breech presentation. Obstetrical complications
2.4 Complete unilateral vaginal or cervico-vaginal atresia with communicating uteri	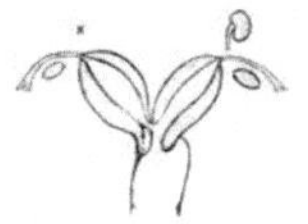	Bicornis-unicollis uterus with an anomalous horn and ipsilateral RA	No symptoms Reproductive Breech presentation Obstetrical complications
2.5 Idem, without communicating uteri	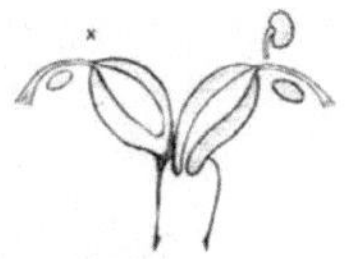	Unicornuate uterus with contralateral unattached but cavitated rudimentary horn URA	Pain. Increasing dysmenorrhea after surgery? Symptoms as endometriosis
3. Isolated or common uterine or utero-vaginal anomalies, affecting			
A. Paramesonephric or müllerian ducts			
A.1. Agenesis or hypoplasias	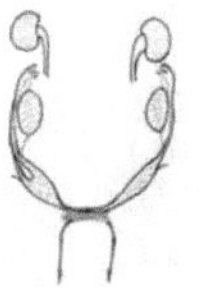	Müllerian agenesis	Primary amenorrhoea Endometriosis and criptomenorrhea if cavitated horn
A.2. Unicornuate uterus with atretic cavitated or non-cavitated rudimentary horn, or segmentary atresia, or 'unilateral Rokitansky syndrome'	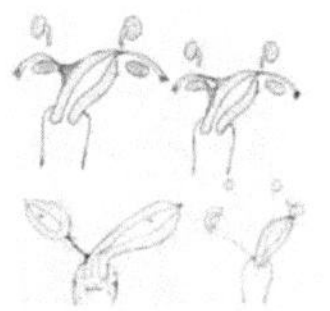	Unicornuate uterus; or bicornuate with cavitated noncommunicated uterine horn or segmentary atresia	Reproductive. Breech presentation Intra or postmenstrual dysmenorrheal. Endometriosis?

Continued

Fig. 1.3 Acien classification system. *Acien et al. History of Female Genital Tract Hum Reprod 2011. pp 701–703*

Table II *Continued*

Aetiopathogenic anomaly	Anatomical findings	Pathology name	Clinical symptoms
A.3. Didelphys uterus	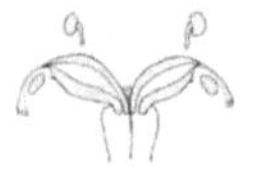	Didelphys uterus	Reproductive Breech presentation
A.4. Bicornuate uterus. Eventually, with a non-communicating cavitated uterine horn	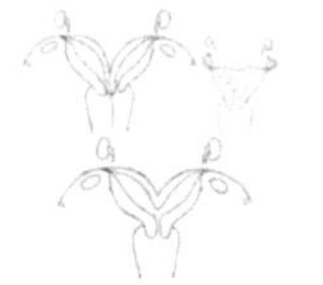	Bicornis-bicollis uterus and Bicornis-unicollis uterus (non-communicating cavitated horn)	Reproductive Miscarriage. Breech presentation Inmature delivery. Retrograde menstruation
A.5. Septate uterus	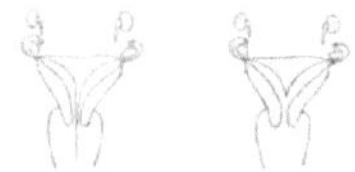	Septate and subseptate uterus	Reproductive Miscarriage Breech presentation Inmature and premature delivery
A.6. Arcuate uterus	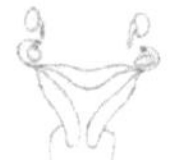	Arcuate uterus	Reproductive losses?
A.7. Anomalies related to DES syndrome	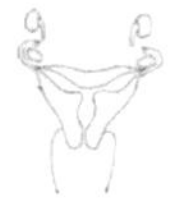	DES syndrome. Hypoplastic and T-shaped uterus. Tricavitated uterus	Infertility Reproductive losses
B. Müllerian tubercle B.1. Complete vaginal or cervico-vaginal agenesis or atresia		Vaginal or cervico-vaginal atresia	Primary amenorrhoea Pain Cryptomenorrhea. Endometriosis
B.2. Segmentary atresias	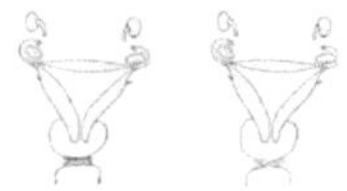	Complete or incomplete transverse vaginal septum	Dyspareunia? Obstetrical problems? Or primary amenorrhoea and cryptomennorrhea
C. Both Müllerian tubercle and ducts Complete utero-vaginal agenesis		Rokitansky or MRKH syndrome	Primary amenorrhoea
4. Accesory uterine masses and other gubernaculum dysfunctions	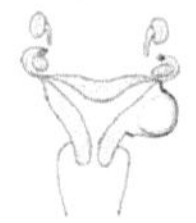	Accesory and cavitated uterine masses with normal uterus. Didelphic uterus without RA?	Pain Dysmenorrhea Tumor
5. Anomalies of the urogenital sinus	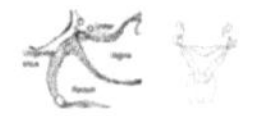	Imperforated hymen. Persistent urogenital sinus. Congenital vesico-vaginal fistula.	Cryptomenorrhea Pain Menuria, Hypospadias, Cloacal fistulas

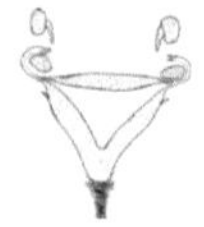

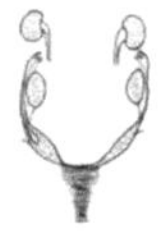

Continued

Table II *Continued*

Aetiopathogenic anomaly	Anatomical findings	Pathology name	Clinical symptoms
6. Malformative combinations	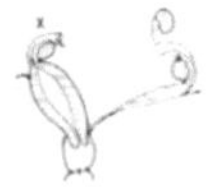	Variable	Variable

URA, unilateral renal agenesis; RA, renal agenesis; MRKH, Mayer–Rokitansky–Kuster–Hauser; DES, diethylstilbestrol.

Fig. 1.3 (continued)

TABLE 1

Description of the individual malformations relative to the organ.

Vagina (V)	0	Normal
	1a	Partial hymenal atresia
	1b	Complete hymenal atresia
	2a	Incomplete septate vagina <50%
	2b	Complete septate vagina
	3	Stenosis of the introitus
	4	Hypoplasia
	5a	Unilateral atresia
	5b	Complete atresia
	S1	Sinus urogenitalis (deep confluence)
	S2	Sinus urogenitalis (middle confluence)
	S3	Sinus urogenitalis (high confluence)
	C	Cloacae
	+	Other
	#	Unknown
Cervix (C)	0	Normal
	1	Duplex cervix
	2a	Unilateral atresia/aplasia
	2b	Bilateral atresia/aplasia
	+	Other
	#	Unknown
Uterus (U)	0	Normal
	1a	Arcuate
	1b	Septate <50% of the uterine cavity
	1c	Septate >50% of the uterine cavity
	2	Bicornate
	3	Hypoplastic uterus
	4a	Unilaterally rudimentary or aplastic
	4b	Bilaterally rudimentary or aplastic
	+	Other
	#	Unknown
Adnexa (A)	0	Normal
	1a	Unilateral tubal malformation, ovaries normal
	1b	Bilateral tubal malformation, ovaries normal
	2a	Unilateral hypoplasia/gonadal streak (including tubal malformation if appropriate)
	2b	Bilateral hypoplasia/gonadal streak (including tubal malformation if appropriate)
	3a	Unilateral aplasia
	3b	Bilateral aplasia
	+	Other
	#	Unknown
associated Malformation (M)	0	None
	R	Renal system
	S	Skeleton
	C	Cardiac
	N	Neurologic
	+	Other
	#	Unknown

Oppelt. VCUAM classification. Fertil Steril 2005.

1494 Oppelt et al. **VCUAM classification** Vol. 84, No. 5, November 2005

Fig. 1.4 VCUAM classification system

ESHRE/ESGE classification
Female genital tract anomalies

Uterine anomaly			Cervical/vaginal anomaly	
Main class	*Sub-class*		*Co-existent class*	
U0 Normal uterus			**C0**	Normal cervix
U1 Dysmorphic uterus	**a.** T-shaped		**C1**	Septate cervix
	b. Infantilis			
	c. Others		**C2**	Double 'normal' cervix
U2 Septate uterus	**a.** Partial		**C3**	Unilateral cervical aplasia
	b. Complete			
			C4	Cervical aplasia
U3 Bicorporeal uterus	**a.** Partial			
	b. Complete			
	c. Bicorporeal septate		**V0**	Normal vagina
U4 Hemi-uterus	**a.** With rudimentary cavity (communicating or not horn)		**V1**	Longitudinal non-obstructing vaginal septum
	b. Without rudimentary cavity (horn without cavity/no horn)		**V2**	Longitudinal obstructing vaginal septum
U5 Aplastic	**a.** With rudimentary cavity (bi- or unilateral horn)		**V3**	Transverse vaginal septum and/or imperforate hymen
	b. Without rudimentary cavity (bi- or unilateral uterine remnants/aplasia)		**V4**	Vaginal aplasia
U6 Unclassified malformations				
U		**C**	**V**	

Associated anomalies of non-Müllerian origin:

Drawing of the anomaly

Figure 3 Scheme for the classification of female genital tract anomalies according to the new ESHRE/ESGE classification system.

Fig. 1.5 The ESHRE-ESGE classification system of mullerian anomalies. *Grimbizis G. The ESHRE/ESGE Consensus. Hum Reprod 2013 p. 2042*

The classification systems all categorize anomalies a little differently which can lead to differences in treatment. For example, when the ESHRE/ESGE criteria was compared to the ASRM classification supplemented with absolute morphometric criteria for the diagnosis of septate uterus, it was found that a significant number of anomalies were categorized as septate by ESHRE/ESGE but considered either arcuate or normal according to the ASRM with additional morphologic criteria [14]. The clinical implication of this discrepancy is that patients would be subjected to surgery when it may not be indicated.

Over the last 100 years, there have been multiple attempts to find a clear, simple, and accurate way to categorize female genital anomalies. All systems appear to have their own strengths and limitations. The simpler classification systems are easier to navigate, but may not adequately capture complex variations while the extensive systems, while more inclusive, are often cumbersome to utilize. However, despite attempts to develop a single inclusive classification system, there are still unique and rare anomalies that often cannot be adequately categorized by the existing systems. Some of the more unusual anomalies are depicted by the following illustrations [7] (Figs. 1.6, 1.7, and 1.8). Clinicians who care for these patients need to be

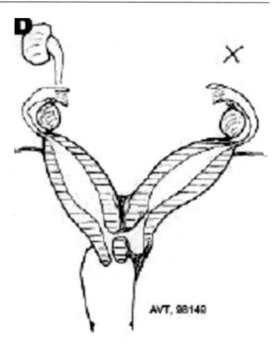

Fig. 1.7 Left cervico-vaginal atresia with bicornuate uterine configuration with communication between left cervico-vaginal area and right hemicervix associated with left renal agenesis. *Acien et al. Hum Reprod. 2004;19:2377–2384*

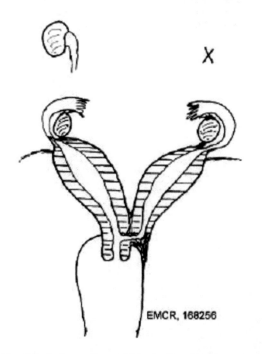

Fig. 1.6 Left cervico-vaginal atresia with bicornuate uterine configuration and communication at the level of cervix. Associated with ipsilateral renal agenesis. *Acien et al. Hum Reprod. 2004;19:2377–2384*

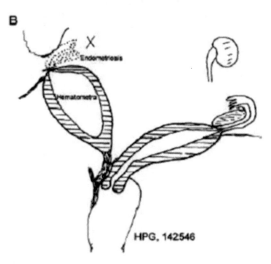

Fig. 1.8 Right obstructed hemiuterus with atretic right hemicervix and normal left hemiuterus and cervix associated with right renal agenesis. *Acien et al. Hum Reprod. 2004;19:2377–2384*

aware that these numerous variations exist and some of these anomalies can be very complex. Sorting out the anatomy correctly is often challenging, and may require "thinking outside the box," but ultimately is important to better facilitate treatment options.

References

1. Strassman P. Die operative vereinigung eines doppelten uterus. Zentralbl Gynaekol. 1907;31:1322.
2. Jones WS. Congenital anomalies of the female genital tract. Trans N Engl Obstet Gynecol Soc. 1953;7: 79–94.
3. Buttram Jr VC, Gibbons WE. Mullerian anomalies: a proposed classification (An analysis of 144 cases). Fertil Steril. 1979;32:40–6.
4. Semmens JP. Congenital anomalies of female genital tract. Functional classification based on review of 56 personal cases and 500 reported cases. Obstet Gynecol. 1962;19:328–50.
5. Green LK, Harris RE. Uterine anomalies. Frequency of diagnosis and associated obstetric complications. Obstet Gynecol. 1976;47:427–9.
6. American Fertility Society. Classification of adnexal adhesions, distal tubal occlusion, tubal occlusion secondary to tubal ligation, tubal pregnancies, Mullerian anomalies, and intrauterine adhesions. Fertil Steril. 1988;49:944–55.
7. Woelfer B, Salim R, Banerjee S, Elson J, Regan L, Jurkovic D. Reproductive outcomes in women with congenital uterine anomalies detected by three-dimensional ultrasound screening. Obstet Gynecol. 2001;98(6):1099–103.
8. Ludwin A, Ludwin I, Banas T, Knafel A, Miedzyblocki M, Basta A. Diagnostic accuracy of sonohysterography, hysterosalpingography and diagnostic hysteroscopy in diagnosis of arcuate, septate and bicornuate uterus. J Obstet Gynaecol Res. 2011;37:178–86.
9. Salim R, Woelfer B, Backos M, Regan L, Jurkovic D. Reproducibility of three dimensional ultrasound diagnosis of congenital uterine anomalies. Ultrasound Obstet Gynecol. 2003;21:578–82.
10. Acien P, Acien M, Sanchez-Ferrer M. Complex malformations of the female genital tract. New types and revision of classification. Hum Reprod. 2004;19: 2377–84.
11. Acien P, Acien MI. The history of female genital tract malformation classifications and proposal of an updated system. Hum Reprod Update. 2011;17: 693–705.
12. Oppelt P, Renner SP, Brucker S, et al. The VCUAM (Vagina Cervix Uterus Adnex-associated Malformation) classification: a new classification for genital malformations. Fertil Steril. 2005;84:1493–7.
13. Grimbizis GF, Gordts S, Di Spiezio SA, et al. The ESHRE/ESGE consensus on the classification of female genital tract congenital anomalies. Hum Reprod. 2013;28:2032–44.
14. Ludwin A, Ludwin I. Comparison of the ESHRE-ESGE and ASRM classifications of Mullerian duct anomalies in everyday practice. Hum Reprod. 2015;30:569–80.

Diagnostic Approach to Müllerian Anomalies

Heather Appelbaum, Jeanne Choi-Rosen, and Shawna Tonick

Introduction

Structural defects of the reproductive tract become apparent at varying chronological times during life and diagnosis may not be straightforward. While congenital anomalies involving the external genitalia are evident at birth, obstructive and nonobstructive Müllerian anomalies may not be recognized in the prepubertal girl unless there are associated defects that raise clinical suspicion. While diagnosis can be made during childhood, congenital anomalies of the Müllerian ducts are more commonly diagnosed in adolescence or later in adult life as an incidental finding during pregnancy or during evaluation for assisted reproduction.

H. Appelbaum, M.D. (✉)
Division of Pediatric and Adolescent Gynecology, Cohen Children's Medical Center of NY/Northwell Medical Center, Hofstra North Shore LIJ School of Medicine, 270-05 76th Ave, New Hyde Park, NY 11040, USA
e-mail: happelba@nshs.edu

J. Choi-Rosen, M.D.
Pediatric Radiology, Cohen Children's Medical Center of NY/Northwell Medical Center, Hofstra North Shore LIJ School of Medicine, 270-05 76th Ave, New Hyde Park, NY 11040, USA

S. Tonick, M.D.
Department of Obstetrics and Gynecology, Cohen Children's Medical Center of NY/Northwell Medical Center, Hofstra North Shore LIJ School of Medicine, 270-05 76th Ave, New Hyde Park, NY 11040, USA

Anomalies of the female reproductive tract result from abnormal development of one or both of the Müllerian ducts, which results in a heterogeneous constellation of symptoms and physical findings. Müllerian malformations may be identified when a patient experiences an array of symptoms including primary amenorrhea; acute, chronic or cyclic pelvic pain; irregular bleeding; foul smelling vaginal discharge; dysmenorrhea; dyspareunia; recurrent spontaneous abortions; cervical incompetence; premature delivery; fetal malposition; or unexplained infertility. Patients with obstructive anomalies are more likely to complain of pain, while nonobstructive anomalies tend to be more asymptomatic. Complex Müllerian anomalies involving one obstructed duct and one patent duct may be difficult to diagnose. These defects present a diagnostic challenge and delay in making the correct diagnosis is not uncommon in early adolescence because pain and irregular bleeding may be attributed to functional or primary dysmenorrhea.

Ultrasound, magnetic resonance imaging (MRI), examination under anesthesia, vaginoscopy, hysteroscopy, laparoscopy, and hysterosalpingogram are all useful tools to define the anatomy so that appropriate management options can be pursued. Obstructive anomalies may require urgent surgical attention to relieve the obstruction, whereas nonobstructive anomalies do not necessarily require surgical intervention unless the patient is adversely affected by the defect.

© Springer International Publishing Switzerland 2016
S.M. Pfeifer (ed.), *Congenital Müllerian Anomalies*, DOI 10.1007/978-3-319-27231-3_2

Primary amenorrhea, dysmenorrhea, or pelvic pain are common causes for referral to the gynecologist. Referrals may involve girls with normal thelarche, pubarche, and growth who have not menstruated. Alternatively, girls with regular or irregular menstrual cycles may present with cyclic abdominal or pelvic pain. In girls with structural abnormalities of the reproductive tract, history and physical examination typically confirm normal progression of these pubertal milestones. In examining the patient, particular attention should be paid to breast development and Tanner staging, the presence of axillary and pubic hair, and careful inspection of the external genitalia and hymenal orifice. Laboratory determinations should be done to confirm normal gonadotropin and sex steroid hormone levels. Karyotype with FISH determination of the SRY gene is useful to understand a discordance between the phenotype and genotype of the individual [1, 2]. Further genetic screening may be indicated in the presence of dysmorphic features suggestive of a genetic syndrome. Imaging studies are essential in all cases to augment the knowledge based on physical findings and clarify the internal reproductive structures. This chapter will provide a comprehensive approach to diagnosis of the structural complexities that can result from congenital anomalies of the reproductive tract. Psychosocial and psychosexual implications related to diagnosis disclosure will be addressed.

History and Physical Examination

Diagnosis of Müllerian anomalies should be based on symptoms, history, and physical examination. Obtaining a clinical history must involve facilitating an open ended discussion with the patient and include menstrual history, bowel and bladder function, sexual activity, pelvic pain, and reproductive history, when relevant. If the patient is a child or adolescent, the parent may provide crucial information pertaining to the medical history of the patient, including results of prenatal testing or imaging identifying developmental issues. Family history of congenital anomalies or infertility should be obtained, as family associations with Müllerian anomalies have been

described. Müllerian anomalies have been suggested to follow multifactorial and polygenic inheritance pattern, with individuals with an affected first degree relative having a 12 times increased risk [3]. A variety of genes are involved in development of the reproductive tract. Mutations of these genes and subsequent transcription factors such as WNT, DACH, HOX, and SOX9 may play a role in abnormal Müllerian duct development (see table from NASPAG committee opinion Obstructive reproductive tract anomalies 12/2014).

Prepubertal Diagnosis

Clinical Presentation of Obstructed Anomalies

Obstructive anomalies in the neonate may present with an abdominal mass and genital examination in the neonate can reveal an imperforate hymen, a persistent urogenital sinus, or a single perineal orifice consistent with a cloacal malformation. Hydrocolpos associated with an obstructed outflow tract may be evident by the presence of an abdominal mass at birth or identified on prenatal ultrasound (Fig. 2.1). When mucocolpos due to an imperforate hymen is present in the neonate a hymenal bulge can be identified (Fig. 2.2). Following withdrawal of maternal hormones, the mucocolpos is absorbed and on careful inspection, only a thin membrane covering the introitus remains. Examination under anesthesia and vaginoscopy using a 9.5 Fr cystoscope can be used to clarify the length of the common channel and associated vaginal malformations in the presence of a persistent urogenital sinus or cloacal malformation (Fig. 2.3a–c). Usage of prenatal ultrasound and MRI has been described in the evaluation of disorders of sex development and hydrocolpos although there are no large series that specifically address diagnosis of Müllerian anomalies using prenatal imaging [4, 5]. Nevertheless, as technology advances and with increasing access and performance of fetal MRIs, the application of prenatal imaging to diagnose Müllerian abnormalities will continue to evolve.

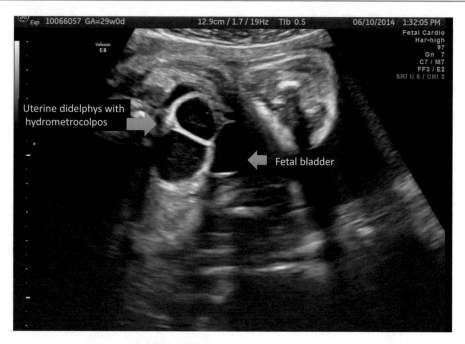

Fig. 2.1 Prenatal ultrasound identifying duplicated vagina with hydrocolpos (Courtesy of Natalie Meirowitz, M.D.)

Obstructive Müllerian defects that are identified early allow for intervention prior to the onset of menarche and possible prevention of potential complications associated with later diagnosis in adolescence including pelvic pain associated with hematocolpos, constipation and/or urinary retention, endometriosis, pelvic inflammatory disease, ectopic pregnancies, and fertility compromise [6].

Clinical Presentation of Nonobstructed Anomalies

Nonobstructive variations in anatomy of the uterus and vagina are commonly asymptomatic and generally are not associated with abnormalities of the external genitalia. As a result, these defects in Müllerian duct development are not typically diagnosed before puberty. Routine physical examination would not reveal an isolated Müllerian anomaly and therefore when diagnosis is made in the young girl it is usually in association with other malformations or as an incidental radiologic or surgical finding.

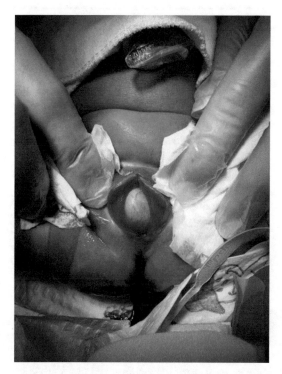

Fig. 2.2 Neonatal imperforate hymen with mucocolpos (Courtesy of Elana Kastner, M.D.)

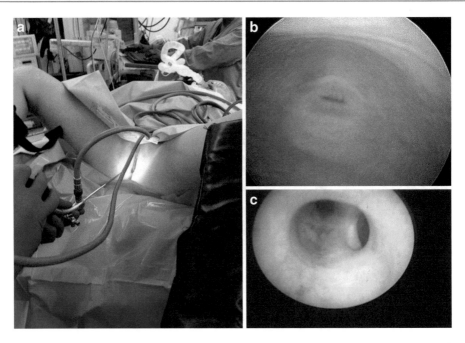

Fig. 2.3 (**a**) Vaginoscopy and examination under anesthesia with 9.5 fr cystoscope. (**b**) Vaginsocopy showing normal vagina and cervix at apex. (**c**) Common channel in persistent urogenital sinus (Courtesy of Heather Appelbaum, M.D.)

Urinary tract abnormalities are the most common abnormality associated with congenital anomalies of the reproductive tract. Simultaneous embryologic development of the paramesonephros and the metanephros results in 30–50 % association of Müllerian anomalies with renal anomalies [7, 8]. Anomalies include unilateral renal agenesis, duplex collecting systems, horseshoe kidneys, and ectopic or pelvic kidneys. Other associated extragenital malformations include skeletal abnormalities, auditory canal defects, congenital heart disease, inguinal hernias, and anorectal malformations. Vertebral and non-vertebral skeletal abnormalities can be seen in approximately 7–44 % of patients; cardiac defects and ear related anomalies have been reported in up to 25 % of individuals with Müllerian anomalies [9, 10]; Müllerian anomalies have been identified in up to 50 % of individuals with anorectal malformations [11, 12]; and two vessel umbilical cord has also been found to be associated with these anomalies [13]. The diagnosis of one or more of these related abnormalities should raise clinical suspicion for a Müllerian anomaly and prompt investigation of the Müllerian structures.

Postpubertal Diagnosis

If a Müllerian defect is not detected in early childhood, diagnosis is typically delayed until adolescence at the time of puberty, during the sexual debut of the adolescent or young adult patient, or when reproductive complications arise. A timeline of breast, pubic, and axillary hair development and growth history should be obtained. Generally, menarche occurs 2 years following thelarche and correlates with a Tanner stage 3–4 breast development. Patients should be evaluated 3 years post thelarche or at age 15 years if menarche has not occurred in the setting of normal secondary sexual development [14, 15]. Examination technique should begin with inspection and Tanner staging should be determined. Confidentiality and privacy should be considered at the time of examination of adolescents. Abdominal examination is required to assess for tenderness and/or the presence of a suprapubic or abdominal mass. Genital examination techniques may vary depending on the individual patient. Most patients can be examined in the lithotomy position. Frog legged or knee to chest

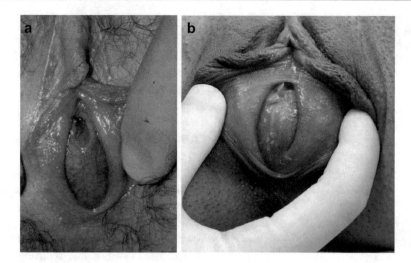

Fig. 2.4 (**a**) Classic "blue-hued bulge" with valsalva representing build op of menstrual fluid distending the thin hymen at the introitus. (**b**) Bulge at the hymen with valsalva. Note the hymen is thicker in this case so does not appear as "blue" (Courtesy of Heather Appelbaum, M.D.)

positioning can be used for smaller children. Gentle traction on the labia majora allows for adequate inspection of the hymen. An imperforate hymen will protrude with Valsalva maneuvering or with application of pressure to a suprapubic mass (Fig. 2.4a, b). Alternatively, a cotton tipped applicator can be used to assess the hymenal structure and is particularly useful to evaluate the length and caliber of the vaginal canal or a vaginal dimple in non-sexually active girls. A speculum examination is generally avoided in girls that are not sexually active unless the examination is performed under anesthesia. Alternatively, vaginoscopy can be performed under anesthesia with a 9.5 Fr cystoscope to allow for adequate, complete, and atraumatic visualization of the urogenital structures including the bladder, vagina, and cervix (Fig. 2.3a). The urethra, perineum, and anus should be inspected. Digital rectal exam is equally, or more, invasive than a vaginal examination and is not well tolerated in younger patients and the authors' opinion is that it should be avoided, unless performed under anesthesia.

Primary Amenorrhea without Abdominal Pain

Agenesis of the uterus, cervix, and vagina (Müllerian agenesis) is the second most common cause of primary amenorrhea and is the most common structural defect resulting in primary amenorrhea without pelvic or abdominal pain. Alternative causes of primary amenorrhea must be considered including hypothalamic amenorrhea, ovulatory dysfunction, constitutional delay, ovarian failure, and other endocrine imbalances or aberrant pharmacologic or environmental exposures including chemotherapeutic agents or radiation [14]. Nutritional status and caloric intake together with energy expenditure should be assessed. Psychosocial and/or psychosexual issues should be addressed including sexual maturity and when addressing adolescents, high risk behaviors associated with the likelihood of sexual activity should be discussed confidentially with the patient in absence of the parent or legal guardian [16].

Müllerian agenesis, also known as Mayer-Rokitansky-Küster-Hauser (MRKH) syndrome, occurs in 1 of 4–5000 live female births [17]. Individuals with MRKH have a 46 XX karyotype. Because ovarian function is unaffected in girls with MRKH, pubertal onset and development of secondary sexual characteristics is unaffected. On physical examination, normal breast development and pubic hair is evident. Pelvic examination identifies normal external genitalia and hymenal structure. A cotton tipped applicator can be used to identify vagina mucosa proximal to the hymen but the vaginal canal is absent

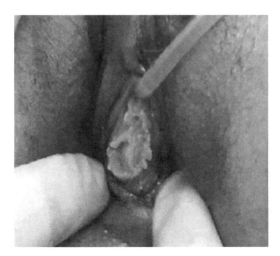

Fig. 2.5 External genital exam showing normal hymenal tissue with blind ending vagina (Courtesy of Heather Appelbaum, M.D.)

(Fig. 2.5). This should not be confused with an imperforate hymen or distal transverse septum.

Other conditions associated with Müllerian duct aplasia include Müllerian-renal-cervical syndrome (MURCS), Klippel-Feil, Fraser syndrome, and some anorectal malformation. Certain disorders of sexual differentiation may have varying degrees of associated Müllerian or vaginal agenesis including mixed gonadal dysgenesis, complete androgen insensitivity syndrome (CAIS), or partial androgen sensitivity syndrome (PAIS). Chromosomal studies and testosterone levels are important to help differentiate between these complex diagnoses. Individuals with CAIS have a 46 XY karyotype, but appear phenotypically as normal females. Individuals with CAIS have an androgen receptor defect that prevents appropriate cellular and organ developmental responses to testosterone and dihydrotestosterone. The gene for androgen receptor expression is located on the X chromosome, and therefore this condition may be inherited as an X-linked condition or associated with a sporadic mutation. Estrogen is produced as a result of aromatization of testosterone with resulting normal expression of estrogen response related pubertal changes including breast development. Secondary sexual hair growth is scanty or absent in these individuals due to the defective androgen receptor. The external examination is invariably female in individuals with CAIS. The vagina is generally under developed but may have more length than girls with MRKH, whereas girls with PAIS may have ambiguous features due to some androgen effect on the external genitalia.

Amenorrhea and Pelvic Pain

Obstructive Müllerian defects result in impediment of menstrual egress and subsequent development of hematocolpos or hematometrocolpos. The obstruction can involve the hymen, vagina, cervix, or uterine horn. Patients present initially with episodic dysmenorrhea that typically progresses to worsening or constant pelvic pain. The cyclic or intermittent pain increases with each cycle and ultimately may become so intense that the patient presents with an acute emergency secondary to severe and debilitating pelvic pain, urinary retention, or constipation. In severe cases, a grossly distended vagina can cause a mechanical obstruction of the ureter resulting in hydronephrosis.

With an imperforate hymen the vagina is not affected structurally. Therefore accumulated menstrual blood can cause significant vaginal distention leading to a large pelvic/abdominal mass and associated severe pelvic or abdominal pain, urinary retention, or constipation. Abdominal examination may identify a large tender suprapubic mass, which may extend to above the umbilicus, while visual inspection of the vulva reveals a hymenal membrane that is bulging (Fig. 2.4a, b). Valsalva maneuvering or gentle pressure on the suprapubic mass intensifies the hymenal bulge of an imperforate hymen when the hymenal examination is equivocal. Imaging by ultrasound, CT scan, or MRI will reveal a large hematocolpos with the obstruction extending low down to the level of the pelvic symphysis (Fig. 2.6a–c).

Similarly, a transverse vaginal septum can present with amenorrhea and cyclic pelvic pain associated with a pelvic mass. However, depending on the size of the upper vagina, these girls present with symptoms earlier than those with an imperforate hymen because the vagina cannot distend as easily. Girls with a transverse vaginal septum have a normal hymenal opening but a short vagina.

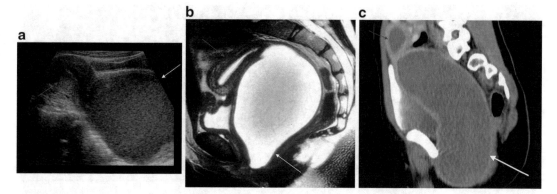

Fig. 2.6 Imaging of imperforate hymen: (**a**) US, (**b**) MRI, and (**c**) CT. *Red arrow* points to uterus, *white arrow* points to hematocolpos. Note the large hematocolpos that extends to below the symphysis on both MRI and CT images (Courtesy of Jeanne Choi-Rosen, M.D.)

Vaginal depth varies with the location of the septum. Segmental vaginal agenesis is a rare obstructive defect where the vagina or a portion of the lower vagina is aplastic or atretic but the upper vagina, cervix, and the uterus are appropriately developed, thus leading to a similar presentation of cyclic abdominal pain and amenorrhea associated with a pelvic mass (Fig. 2.7a–c). The hymen is normal in appearance and the vagina appears absent. Cervical agenesis presents in a similar fashion, although the vagina is usually present, but blind ended and non-communicating with the uterus and there is no vaginal or hymenal bulging.

Pelvic ultrasound may be sufficient to assess uncomplicated Müllerian anomalies. In contrast, complex anomalies must be further evaluated by pelvic MRI to assess the degree and exact location of the defect to allow for adequate surgical planning. MRI is considered superior to pelvic ultrasound for evaluation of combined vertical and lateral defects as the images provide clear delineation of uterine, cervical, and vaginal anatomy in multiple imaging planes (Figs. 2.6 and 2.7). MRI may not be able to clearly diagnose specific subtle cervical architectural abnormalities or other rare variations of Müllerian duct development. Complex anomalies may require diagnostic laparoscopy to resolve diagnostic uncertainties [18]. Referral should be made to a tertiary care center with specific expertise in congenital anomalies of the reproductive tract for accurate diagnosis and appropriate surgical intervention [19, 20]. Hormonal suppressive

therapy should be provided if treatment delay is necessary. Foley catheter insertion may be indicated to ameliorate urinary retention. Needle aspiration or drainage of hematocolpos should not be attempted as this can introduce bacteria into a closed and sterile environment and may lead to severe pelvic inflammatory disease or sepsis [21]. Complications such as endometriosis, pelvic abscess, chronic pelvic pain, or infertility associated with outflow tract obstructions may be prevented with surgical intervention to restore the conduit for menstrual egress.

Pelvic Pain Associated with Menstruation

Patients with a duplicated Müllerian system may have a complex configuration where one Müllerian duct is patent while the contralateral side is non-communicating. Menstruation occurs through the patent side. However, on the obstructed side, menstrual blood will accumulate above the level of obstruction, leading to pain and, depending on the level of obstruction, development of a mass (hematocolpos or hematometra). One of the more common conditions associated with this scenario is double uterus with obstructed hemivagina. This anomaly is usually seen in combination with ipsilateral renal agenesis and is known as "obstructed hemivagina and ipsilateral renal agenesis" (OHVIRA) or Herlyn-Werner-Wunderlich Syndrome (HWW)

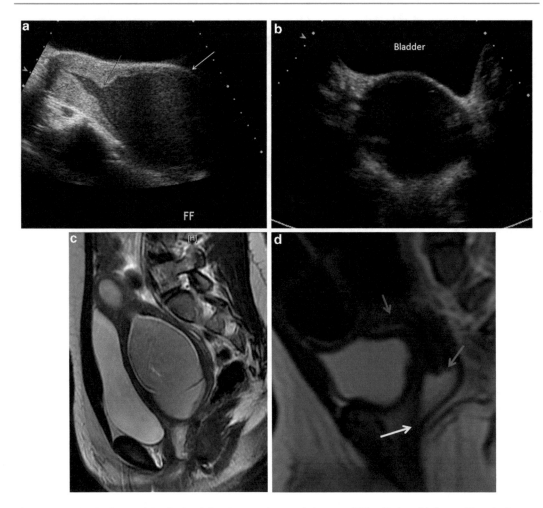

Fig. 2.7 (a) Sagittal transabdominal pelvic ultrasound imaging of patient with distal vaginal agenesis showing hematometra and distended cervix. *Red line* points to dilated cervix. *White line* points to the hematocolpos. (b) Transverse transabdominal pelvic ultrasonographic imaging of distended vagina. (c) MRI showing distal vaginal agenesis. The cervix is not well identified on this image. Note the hematocolpos does not extend as far inferiorly as one would see with an imperforate hymen. (d) Sagittal T2 weighted image. Note the uterus (*red arrow*), cervix (*blue arrow*), and hydrocolpos (*yellow arrow*) in this patient with distal vaginal atresia (Courtesy of Jeanne Choi-Rosen, M.D.)

[22]. With this condition, the uterus may be didelphic or complete septate configuration. Girls with OHVIRA present shortly after menarche with regular or irregular periods and progressive dysmenorrhea that does not respond well to pain medications or cyclic hormonal therapy. These girls menstruate from the patent tract but simultaneously develop hematocolpos with or without hematometra on the obstructed side (Fig. 2.8a–c). Cyclic pelvic pain associated with menses may progress to constant pelvic pain and the pelvic mass resulting from accumu-lation of blood can effectively compromise rectal capacity leading to constipation. Similarly, bladder capacity may be affected and frequency of urination, urinary retention, or hydronephrosis can ensue from compression of the urinary tract. A tender suprapubic mass can be palpated on physical exam and an asymmetric bulging of the lateral vaginal wall may be visible or palpable on pelvic examination (Fig. 2.9). A cotton tipped applicator can be used to demonstrate a unilateral patent vagina. Rarely in individuals with OHVIRA the obstruction may be at the

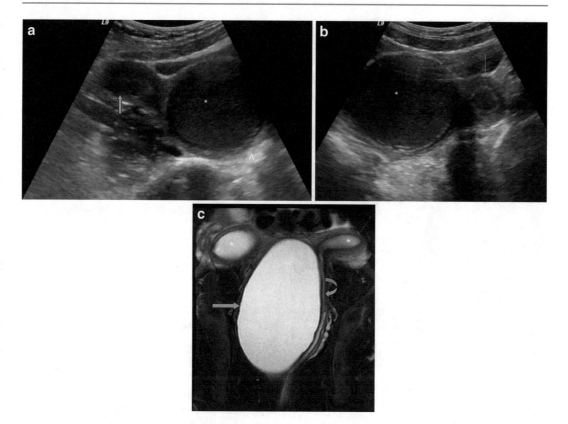

Fig. 2.8 Uterine didelphys with obstructed left hemivagina. (**a**) Transabdominal sonogram with normal right uterine horn (*arrow*) and hematocolpos (*asterisk*). (**b**) Transabdominal image in transverse with hematometra (*arrow*) and hematocolpos (*asterisk*). (**c**) MRI Coronal T2 weighted image showing uterus didelphys with distended *right* hematocolpos (*arrow*). The right uterine horn (*asterisk*) is distended with blood. The left uterine horn (*asterisk*) is normal. The left hemivagina is normal and seen coursing adjacent to the right hematocolpos (*curved arrow*). MRI offers advantage of visualizing both uterine horns and distended vagina in one image (Courtesy of Jeanne Choi-Rosen, M.D.)

level of the cervix rather than vagina, but also associated with unilateral renal agenesis [18].

Rarely, patients present with regular menses and significant menstrual spotting that can last for days to weeks after the end of the regular menstrual period. If the patient has a double uterus, either uterus didelphys or a complete septate uterus, then there may be a microperforation between the obstructed and nonobstructed side at the level of the vagina, cervix, or uterus. The microperforation may not be apparent on exam or imaging. Alternatively, pyocolpos may develop in the obstructed side due to an ascending vaginal infection [23]. In this case the individual will present with copious foul smelling vaginal discharge that typi-

cally does not respond to traditional antibiotic therapy for vaginitis.

Alternatively, girls with unicornuate uteri and contralateral functional rudimentary uterine horns can develop hematometra in the non-communicating uterine horn. This complex defect can present with unilateral cyclic abdominal pain associated with menstruation that is refractory to pain medications or hormonal treatments. With this condition, there is not usually a large pelvic mass and the uterine horn does not distend significantly. Occasionally, a pelvic collection, pelvic infection, or even hemodynamic instability from a ruptured ectopic pregnancy may be the first evidence of a functional noncommunicating uterine horn [24, 25]. Vulvar and

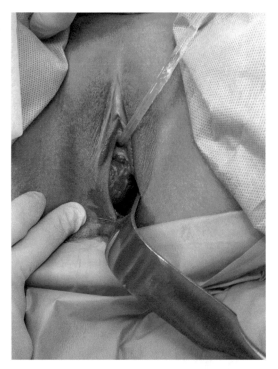

Fig. 2.9 Bulging of the right lateral vaginal wall associated with a right obstructed hemivagina (Courtesy of Heather Appelbaum, M.D.)

vaginal examinations are normal in patients with an obstructed uterine horn as the functional uterine horn is associated with the presence of a single cervix at the vaginal apex. MRI of the pelvis is helpful to confirm diagnosis (Fig. 2.10).

Vaginal Anomalies

Vaginal anomalies can present with pain with tampon insertion or dyspareunia or they can go undiagnosed for years. A microperforate transverse vaginal septum may allow for menstrual egress, but limits the caliber of the vagina resulting in pain with coitus or inability to insert tampons. On examination, the cervix cannot be visualized and generally is nonpalpable. Noncircumferential vaginal bands of fibrous tissue within the vaginal rugae in the transverse plane are a form of incomplete transverse septum that my result in pain with coital activity because of the inability of this abnormal tissue to stretch with pressure [20]. A longitudinal vaginal septum may be com-

pletely asymptomatic, present as failure for tampons "to work," or also present with dyspareunia (Fig. 2.11). The septum can be a cause of pain if direct pressure is applied to a midline septum or penetration of an asymmetric atretic vagina is attempted. Furthermore, trauma to the septum can occur with intercourse resulting in pain and/or hemorrhage (Fig. 2.12). A longitudinal vaginal septum may result in complaints related to tampon insertion associated with discomfort or incomplete menstrual hygiene because of menstrual blood loss through the side of the vagina not containing the tampon [20].

Reproductive Complications

Nonobstructive Müllerian anomalies are commonly asymptomatic anatomical findings that are incidentally diagnosed during physical examination, during surgical or radiologic evaluation of other disorders, or even at time of cesarean section. Speculum examination may reveal an asymptomatic longitudinal vaginal septum and/or cervical duplication (Fig. 2.11). Alternatively, diagnosis of various Müllerian defects via ultrasound, 3D ultrasound, or hysterosalpingogram may occur at the time of an investigation for causes of infertility or miscarriage.

Nonobstructed Müllerian anomalies which allow for normal menstrual egress and are not associated with pelvic pain generally remain asymptomatic but may cause complications associated with pregnancy. Asymptomatic uterine anomalies such as bicornuate, septate, didelphys, and unicornuate uteri are more typically diagnosed due to adverse pregnancy outcomes and compromised fertility. These isolated defects may be associated with spontaneous abortion, recurrent abortions, preterm labor, fetal malposition, labor abnormalities, or low birth weight. Diminished uterine capacity found in patients with uterine didelphys or unicornuate uterus leads to fetal malposition, preterm delivery, and lower birth weight at term, and increased risk of pregnancy loss [20]. Complications related to labor and delivery are increased in women with Müllerian anomalies. Cesarean delivery rate is

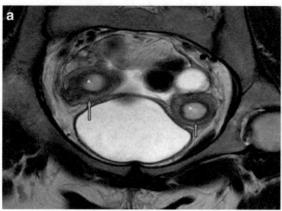

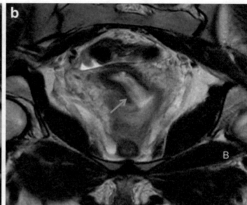

Fig. 2.10 Obstructed left uterine horn. (**a**) Coronal T2 weighted image showing with two widely separate uterine horns (*asterisk*). Note both have dark T2 signal of the junctional zone present (*arrows*). (**b**) Only the right uter- ine horn had a cervix (*arrow*) and communicated with the vagina. The left rudimentary uterine horn did not com- municate and there was no cervix identified (Courtesy of Jeanne Choi-Rosen, M.D.)

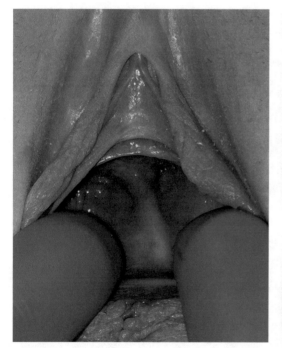

Fig. 2.11 Longitudinal vaginal septum (Courtesy of Heather Appelbaum, M.D.)

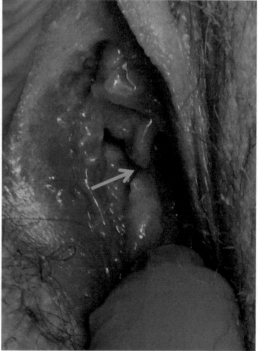

Fig. 2.12 Traumatic rupture of longitudinal vaginal septum (Courtesy of Heather Appelbaum, M.D.)

increased secondary to fetal malposition or labor dystocia in patients with vaginal septums [26, 27]. Laceration and bleeding of vaginal septum may lead to intrapartum hemorrhage. Separated uteri are associated with higher risk of preterm birth, spontaneous pregnancy loss, and fetal malpresentation [27]. Speculation has been made that these adverse outcomes may be due to poor vascularization of the septum or poor pla- centation for pregnancies that implant on the septum [28]. Intervention may be undertaken to restore the uterine cavity to normal anatomy which may enhance pregnancy outcome [29–31]. Interestingly, in most studies arcuate uterus is not associated with adverse pregnancy outcomes [26, 27, 31], but recent meta-analysis has shown that there may be an association with fetal malposition and increased pregnancy loss [32].

Diagnostic Imaging

Anatomical abnormalities of the female reproductive tract can be further delineated with pelvic imaging and pelvic imaging is an important part of the diagnostic process. Precise radiologic diagnosis is necessary to guide surgical intervention and is imperative for appropriate fertility counseling. Transabdominal, transvaginal, transrectal, transperineal, and 3D ultrasound have all been used to clarify the anatomy when an anomaly is suspected. Pelvic ultrasound is the preferred initial imaging modality. MRI is considered the gold standard for diagnosis of Müllerian anomalies and is used to assess the length of the vagina, the thickness of a septum, and to delineate the configuration and number of the cervix or cervices and uterus or uteri. MRI is particularly helpful to assess communication between Müllerian structures and is essential to determine the presence of a functional endometrium in rudimentary uterine horns (Fig. 2.10). MRI is especially useful in evaluating complex Müllerian anomalies and should be used to guide surgical management. Hysterosalpingogram (HSG) with the use of fluoroscopy can be used to assess endometrial shape and tubal patency in nonobstructive uterine anomalies, such as septate, bicornuate, and unicornuate uteri (Fig. 2.13). In addition, HSG can also be used to assess communication between uteri, cervices, and vaginas in the case of a duplicated Müllerian anomaly when a microperforation or communication is suspected. In the adolescent HSG is typically performed under anesthesia at the time of diagnostic evaluation such as exam under anesthesia, vaginoscopy, and cystoscopy. Diagnostic laparoscopy or hysteroscopy has been considered the gold standard for the diagnosis of Müllerian anomalies as the inner and outer uterine contour

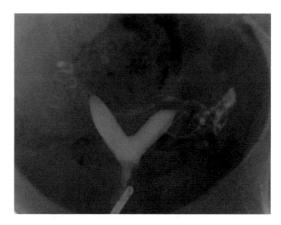

Fig. 2.13 Hysterosalpingogram of partial septate uterus. Note that the HSG identifies two endometrial cavities but cannot differentiate between septate and bicornuate uterus (*Image provided by David E Reichman M.D.*)

can be assessed simultaneously. However, radiologic imaging is becoming the preferred diagnostic modality due to greater accuracy with the advances in technology of MRI, ultrasound, and 3D ultrasound, and because these techniques are less invasive than surgical approaches [33]. However, combined diagnostic laparoscopy and hysteroscopy/vaginoscopy are still valuable tools in diagnosing and classifying Müllerian anomalies for the infertile patient [34] but more importantly in the adolescent with a complex anomaly to augment information obtained through imaging and to facilitate diagnosis and better formulate a treatment plan.

Transabdominal Ultrasound

Transabdominal sonography is the most common initial imaging modality of the female pelvis in the pediatric/adolescent population as well as in adults. The exam is most often performed utilizing a distended urinary bladder as an acoustic window. A distended bladder helps to displace air containing bowel loops that can impede the ability to visualize the pelvic structures. Which transducer to use to best image the pelvis will depend on the patient's body habitus and age. For very young patients, including neonates, a curved array 8-5 MHz transducer or high frequency linear

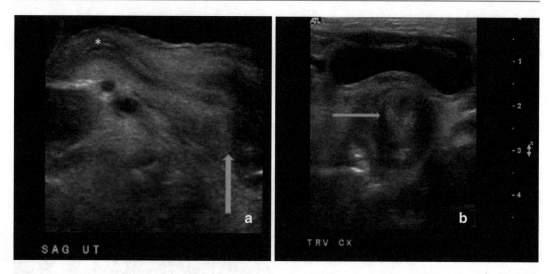

Fig. 2.14 Neonatal transabdominal pelvic ultrasound emphasizing a prominent cervix. The shape of the neonatal uterus has been described as spade shaped, tube shaped, and pear shaped. (**a**) Sagittal view demonstrating "spade shape" where the cervix (*arrow*) is more prominent than the fundus (*asterisk*). (**b**) Transverse image of the cervix (Courtesy of Jeanne Choi-Rosen, M.D.)

transducer such as a 12-5 MHz may be ideal. For young children, the curved array 8-5 MHz transducer is often sufficient. For older children and those with large body habitus where deeper penetration of sound waves is necessary, a curved 5-1 MHz transducer is recommended [35].

Imaging of the pelvis is performed in both the sagittal and transverse planes. Often, the transducer will need to be angled in order to obtain the ideal sagittal and transverse images. The images should be obtained in the midline of the structure of interest and extend to each lateral aspect when scanning in the sagittal plane, and several images from cephalad to caudad in the transverse plane. One advantage of the newer sonography units is the ability to record cine loop images, which allows those images of the pelvis to be reviewed as a dynamic scan. While the transabdominal approach allows for a noninvasive assessment of the pelvic organs, the distance of the structures from the skin surface can limit optimal tissue contrast from being achieved, often requiring further imaging to fully delineate the pelvic structures. Bowel gas can often obscure visualization of the pelvic organs as well.

It is important that the imager be well acquainted with the different appearance of the pelvic organs at different ages [35–37]. In the neonate, the uterus and cervix are prominent due to in utero maternal hormonal stimulation (Fig. 2.14a, b). As a result, the echogenic endometrium can often be appreciated during the early neonatal period. In the immediate neonatal period, the cervix is more prominent than the uterus. In the absence of hormonal stimulation, infants and children typically have a tubular configuration to the uterus and cervix, and the uterus and cervix are generally comparable in width (Fig. 2.15). Furthermore, it is difficult to appreciate the endometrium in a non-stimulated child. A prepubertal uterus should not be confused with an underdeveloped or rudimentary uterus. The pubertal or postpubertal uterus is like that of the adult, with the uterine fundus more prominent than the cervix and the echogenic endometrium can again be appreciated, while the thickness varies with the menstrual cycle (Fig. 2.16a) [36].

Sonocolpography to better assess vaginal anomalies such as a transverse septum has been described. A catheter with a balloon is placed within the vagina and transabdominal sonogram is performed to assess the relationship of the vagina to the remainder of the visualized pelvic organs [38].

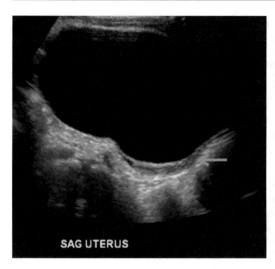

Fig. 2.15 After the neonatal period the uterus has a more tubular shape (*arrow*) (Courtesy of Jeanne Choi-Rosen, M.D.)

Transvaginal Ultrasound

Transvaginal ultrasound is a very useful diagnostic tool for imaging the female pelvis in girls who are sexually active. Unlike transabdominal sonography, it is performed with an empty bladder using an endocavitary C10-4ec Mhz transducer. The endocavitary probe is lubricated and then a condom is placed over the probe. Any air around the probe within the condom should be expressed and then the condom is lubricated and the probe is inserted into the vagina. The patient should be placed in the lithotomy position for the examination. Alternatively, the pelvis can be tilted with a bolster under the buttocks and the knees flexed. When possible, it may be more comfortable and decrease anxiety to have the patient to gently insert the probe herself. A properly positioned transvaginal probe should not be abutting the cervix and should not hurt [35].

The advantage of the transvaginal technique is better tissue delineation because the probe is closer to the pelvic structures. Tissue contrast is significantly more superior using this technique when compared with the transabdominal approach to imaging pelvic anatomy (Fig. 2.16b). Endovaginal ultrasound is the preferred modality in the adolescent and adult population but should not be performed in children or non-sexually active adolescents or adults.

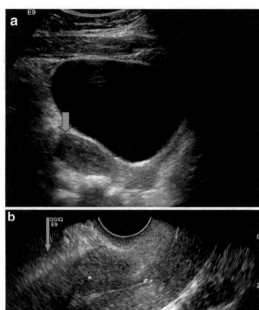

Fig. 2.16 (**a**) Transabdominal sagittal ultrasound image of the postpubertal uterus. Note the fundus is prominent (*arrow*). (**b**) Transvaginal sagittal ultrasound image of the postpubertal uterus. Note again the fundus is prominent (*arrow*). The bright echogenic endometrial canal is also better appreciated (*asterisk*) (Courtesy of Jeanne Choi-Rosen, M.D.)

Transperineal Ultrasound

A transperineal window may supplement images obtained from a transabdominal or transvaginal approach, providing additional information such as the distance between the perineal surface and an obstructed vagina. It is often performed with a high frequency linear transducer however, on occasion a curved array transducer may be utilized if the structure of interest is deeper to the skin surface than a higher frequency transducer can visualize. The probe is lubricated and then covered and then more coupling gel is applied over the covering before the probe is placed on the perineum. Ideally images should be obtained in orthogonal planes and surrounding structures clearly delineated [39].

Transrectal Ultrasound

Transrectal sonography has been described in children and adolescents to facilitate imaging of the pelvis when a transvaginal approach is not feasible [40]. It is performed in a manner similar to the transvaginal exam. The probe is covered in gel and then covered by a plastic sheath. Air around the probe is expressed and then the probe and sheath lubricated and placed within the rectum. In one series of 42 patients, the most common application of the transrectal sonogram was for placement of drainage catheters for deep pelvic collections amenable to transrectal drainage [41]. Fedele et al. described 9 patients where transrectal sonography was performed during the preoperative assessment of congenital vaginal canalization defects [42]. The authors concluded that transrectal ultrasonography is superior to transabdominal and transvaginal ultrasonography in the evaluation of vaginal canalization anomalies, particularly when transvaginal approach is not feasible as in girls with absent vagina. Furthermore, the image definition of transrectal ultrasound allows for more accurate visualization of structures cranial to the imperforate portion of the vagina in girls with incomplete vaginas. Transrectal ultrasound may be limited by patient comfort level with this endocavitary approach.

3D Ultrasound

3D sonography of the female pelvis has been described in the adult literature using an endovaginal probe. It has been shown to be helpful in evaluation of pelvic masses, congenital anomalies of the uterus, and pelvic floor dysfunction. It has potential to be useful for evaluation of congenital reproductive tract anomalies in the pediatric population, although currently there is only literature supporting pediatric 3D imaging in the evaluation of renal and bladder anomalies [43]. In a recent paper by Bermejo et al., excellent correlation with 3D ultrasound and MRI for congenital uterine anomalies (bicornuate, septate, didelphic, unicornuate, and arcuate) was demonstrated, although accurate evaluation of the lower uterine and vaginal septal anomalies may be limited [44]. As availability of this type of ultrasound becomes more common in nonobstrectical imaging sites, the utility with respect to evaluation of Müllerian anomalies will increase [45]. Practicality of this imaging modality is limited by the population being studied and the feasibility of using a transvaginal transducer. Data evaluating 3D ultrasound for the evaluation of complex uterine/vaginal anomalies in the adolescent population is lacking.

Contrast enhanced ultrasound is a promising new technology that has been described in evaluation of the kidneys, as well as abdominal and pelvic tumors in children [46]. Further investigation will be required to determine if this technique can be applied to the evaluation of congenital Müllerian anomalies.

Magnetic Resonance Imaging

Magnetic resonance imaging (MRI) is a well-established, excellent diagnostic tool in the evaluation of the female pelvis. MRI delineates structures based on tissue signal characteristics and has a bigger field of view than can be adequately obtained by sonography [47, 48]. Furthermore, images are obtained in multiple planes. Using strong magnetic fields, the hydrogen molecule is excited and its relaxation back to baseline is evaluated and images are produced with the information obtained. Because tissues have different relaxation times, there are characteristic T1 and T2 weighted signals resulting in excellent tissue differentiation, particularly on T2 weighted sequences. T2 weighted imaging is most useful because zonal anatomy of the uterus and vagina can aid in identification of Mullerian structures. Typically, the endometrium has a bright T2 signal, which is surrounded by the low T2 junctional zone and the intermediate signal of the myometrium. A similar pattern is appreciated for the vagina, with the mucosa bright on T2 weighted sequences, the submucosa appearing dark, and the adventitia appearing bright, due to the presence of its venous plexus.

MRI is a noninvasive examination and there is no ionizing radiation involved. Intravenous contrast is generally not required for the examination of noninflammatory structural defects. Newer MRI techniques such as diffusion weighted imaging have been helpful with further delineation of tissue characteristics, although of limited use in the evaluation of congenital anomalies. 3D MRI techniques are being investigated and show promise in pelvic imaging while significantly reducing scan times [49]. Disadvantages of MRI include the need for sedation for younger or claustrophobic patients and limitations related to exam time and cost. It is important that the radiologist is readily available during the scan in order to optimize the plane of imaging as often the pelvic organs may lie in an oblique position relative to the pelvis.

The images should be reviewed by the clinician with the radiologist. Although the American Fertility Society's Classification of Müllerian anomalies is widely used, it has limitations regarding associated vaginal and cervical anomalies. The VCUAM classification is helpful in the imaging evaluation of patients with congenital Müllerian anomalies as it addresses vaginal and adnexal anomalies in addition to uterine abnormalities (see Chap. 1) [50–52]. Anatomical descriptions of the vagina characterizing the vagina as upper (above the bladder base), middle (at the level of the bladder base), and lower (below the bladder base) can further clarify the anatomy. Creighton and Hall-Craggs reported that there is enough confusion to caution clinicians and imagers to strive for more standard terminology between clinical specialties [53]. According to the authors, 8 out of 10 initially discordant findings between MRI and surgery were found to be concordant, and as a result, the authors propose a standard terminology for vaginal anomalies [54]. Hence, it has been recommended that the surgical and radiologic services work closely together to avoid confusion. Interdisciplinary communication between the surgeon and radiologist before and after each case will allow for tailoring specific exam protocols for patients with complex Müllerian anomalies.

Hysterosalpingogram

Hysterosalpingography is used often in fertility evaluations. Hysterosalpingography involves the introduction of radio opaque water soluble contrast via a small catheter into the endometrial canal after placement of a speculum. For congenital anomalies, it is of limited value as it can only opacify a patent lumen and there is no ability to evaluate the uterine fundal contour, which is often important in determining the type of Müllerian anomaly present (Fig. 2.13). Hysterosalpingography can be helpful in the evaluation of the DES exposed uterus, demonstrating the tiny uterine T shape lumen which may not be appreciated on ultrasound or MRI [33]. Hysterosalpingography involves ionizing radiation and requires speculum insertion; therefore, it is not utilized routinely in the younger pediatric population [55]. However, it can be utilized to evaluate patency between duplicated Müllerian structures (vagina, cervix, or uterus) in the case of a complicated anomaly where a communication or microperforation is suspected and is typically performed under anesthesia [56].

There are many options for imaging the female pelvis. Ultrasound is recommended for initial evaluation [35, 50]. However, MRI is an excellent noninvasive imaging technique that allows for greater tissue detail in different imaging planes. As 3D ultrasound technology evolves, it may rival MRI in its use for evaluating uterine anomalies, but its role in the evaluation of complex Müllerian anomalies in the adolescent has yet to be demonstrated. Transrectal ultrasound demonstrates potential promise to delineate the vagina and cervix, perhaps better than currently possible with MRI, but may have limitations in the pediatric/adolescent population as it is more invasive. Hysterosalpingography has a limited role in both the pediatric and adult patient for the evaluation of congenital uterine anomalies and further imaging is required to distinguish the uterine contour in order to differentiate between arcuate, bicornuate, and septated uteri (Fig. 2.17a–c). Computed tomography (CT) does not have any significant advantage over MRI in the evaluation of congeni-

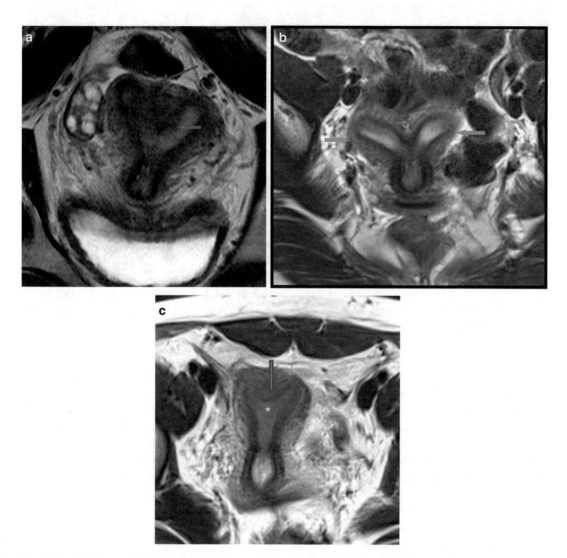

Fig. 2.17 (**a**) Oblique axial T2 weighted MRI image of a septated uterus with a normal fundal contour (*red arrow*) and two endometrial cavities demarcated by a dark T2 signal septation (*arrow*) within the endometrial canal. (**b**) Axial T2 weighted MRI image of a bicornuate uterus with two widely separated uterine horns (*arrows*) and a single cervix (*asterisk*). (**c**) Oblique axial T2 weighted MRI image of an Arcuate uterus. The fundal contour is preserved (*arrow*) with a small, smooth indentation of the endometrial canal (*asterisk*) (Courtesy of Jeanne Choi-Rosen, M.D.)

tal Müllerian anomalies, particularly as it does not have enough tissue contrast to delineate structures, and exposure to ionizing radiation is a considerable disadvantage (Fig. 2.18a–c).

The imaging evaluation of the patient with the congenital anomaly may be tailored based on initial clinical evaluation and sonography. While MRI is the gold standard for evaluating complex Müllerian anomalies, one study spe-

cifically looking at MRKH patients determined that clinical examination and sonography was equally as effective as MRI [51]. Appropriate communication between the surgeon and radiologist and concordance with the terminology to describe the anomalies present will facilitate a clearer understanding of the anatomy. The VCUAM classification is preferred in the imaging evaluation of patients with congenital

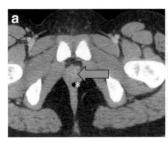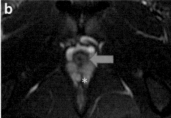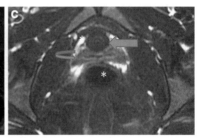

Fig. 2.18 Vaginal agenesis. (**a**) Axial CT scan demonstrating poor tissue contrast between the urethra (*arrow*) and anus (*asterisk*) (**b**) MRI demonstrating absence of the vaginal tissue between the more clearly delineated urethra (*arrow*) and anus (**c**) compared to normal vagina (*curved arrow*) identified on MRI between the urethra (*arrow*) and the anus (*asterisk*) (Courtesy of Jeanne Choi-Rosen, M.D.)

Müllerian anomalies as it addresses vaginal and adnexal anomalies in addition to uterine abnormalities [50–52].

Diagnosis Disclosure

Diagnosis disclosure should be tailored based on the patient's age and level of comprehension, and in a sensitive and descriptive manner. Assessing the patient's cognitive level will allow for more effective disclosure of the anatomical findings and related menstrual, sexual, and reproductive implications. Visual aids including pelvic models or diagrams can be helpful when explaining the anatomy and function of the reproductive organs to patients. Internet health guides and resources are an excellent adjunct to enhance diagnostic awareness; however, these tools should not replace ongoing discussion with the health care provider.

Girls with Müllerian anomalies should be reassured that ovarian function is normal. Therefore, non-syndromic girls with Müllerian anomalies can expect the timing and duration of hormonal changes to be similar to that of the general population. Patients with complex Müllerian anomalies should be counseled on the effect of surgical intervention on sexual functioning and fertility outcomes and referral should be made to a surgeon with expertise in treating these anomalies.

Disclosure of a diagnosis of Müllerian agenesis may result in depression, fear, confusion, or isolation. Concomitant psychosocial intervention is encouraged at the time of initial diagnosis. Ongoing psychosocial support for these young women and their families at each stage of development may help preserve self-image and improve sexual outcomes [57]. Girls with Mullerian agenesis should be further counseled that there are multiple methods of creating a family. Adoption is a well-established process and, in certain circumstances, fertility may be possible using a gestational carrier. New innovations in the field of uterine transplant are currently under investigation. Further research will be necessary to determine candidacy, safety, ethical considerations, and reproductive outcomes [58].

References

1. MacLaughlin DT, Donahoe PK. Sex determination and differentiation. N Engl J Med. 2004;351(3): 306.
2. Lee PA, Houk CP, Ahmed SF, Hughes IA. Consensus statement on management of intersex disorders. Pediatrics. 2006;118(2):e488–500.
3. Hammound AO, Gibson M, Peterson CM, Kerber RA, Mineau G, Hatasaka H. Quantification of the familial contribution to Müllerian anomalies. Obstet Gynecol. 2008;111:378–84.
4. Moshiri M et al. Evaluation and management of disorders of sex development: multidisciplinary approach to a complex diagnosis. Radiographics. 2012;32(6):1599–618.
5. Dhombres F et al. Contribution of prenatal imaging to the anatomical assessment of fetal hydrocolpos. Ultrasound Obstet Gynecol. 2007;30(1):101–4.

6. Fedele L, Bianchi S, Di Nola G, Franchi D, Candiani GB. Endometriosis and nonobstructive Müllerian anomalies. Obstet Gynecol. 1992;79(4):515–7.
7. Oppelt P et al. The VCUAM (Vagina Cervix Uterus Adnexa associated Malformation) classification: a new classification for genital malformations. Fertil Steril. 2005;84(5):1493–7.
8. Sajjad Y. Development of the genital ducts and external genitalia in the early human embryo. J Obstet Gynaecol Res. 2010;36(5):929–37.
9. Kimberley N, Hutson JM, Southwell BR, Grover SR. Vaginal agenesis, the hymen, and associated anomalies. J Pediatr Adolesc Gynecol. 2012;25(1):54–8.
10. Pittock ST, Babovic-Vuksanovic D, Lteif A. Mayer-Rokitansky-Küster-Hauser anomaly and its associated malformations. Am J Med Genet A. 2005;135(3):314–6.
11. Wester T, Tovar JA, Rintala RJ. Vaginal agenesis or distal vaginal atresia associated with anorectal malformations. J Pediatr Surg. 2012;47(3):571–6.
12. Breech LL, Laufer MR. Mullerian anomalies. Obstet Gynecol Clin North Am. 2009;36(1):47–68.
13. Daoub A, Drake TM. Congenital abnormalities of the urogenital tract: the clue is in the cord? BMJ Case Rep. 2014;2014.
14. Practice Committee of the American Society for Reproductive Medicine. Current evaluation of amenorrhea. Fertil Steril. 2008;90(5):S219–25.
15. Emans SJ, Laufer MR, Goldstein DP. Amenorrhea in the adolescent. In: Pediatric and adolescent gynecology. 5th ed. Philadelphia: Lippincott Williams & Wilkins; 2007. p. 214–22.
16. American College of Obstetricians and Gynecologists. Guidelines for adolescent healthcare. 2nd ed. Washington, DC: ACOG; 2011.
17. Chervenak F, Stangel J, Nemee M, Amin H. Mayer Rokitansky Kuster Hauser syndrome. N Y State J Med. 1982;82:23–7.
18. Sabdia S, Sutton B, Kimble RMN. The obstructed hemivagina, ipsilateral renal anomaly, and uterine didelphys triad and the subsequent manifestation of cervical aplasia. J Pediatr Adolesc Gynecol. 2014;27:375–8.
19. Dietrich JE, Millar DM, Quint EH. Non-obstructive Mullerian anomalies. J Pediatr Adolesc Gynecol. 2014;27:386–95.
20. Dietrich JE, Millar DM, Quint EH. Obstructive reproductive tract anomalies. J Pediatr Adolesc Gynecol. 2014;27:396–402.
21. Gidwani G, Falcone T. Congenital malformations of the female genital tract. In: Diagnosis and management. Philadelphia: Lippincott Williams & Wilkins; 1999. p. 145–68.
22. Christianson MS, Yates MM, Woo I, Khafagy A, Garcia JE, Kolp LA. Obstructed Hemivagina Ipsilateral Renal Anomaly (OHVIRA): diagnostic features and management of a frequently misdiagnosed syndrome. Fertil Steril. 2012;98(3):S222.
23. Wozniakowska E. Delayed diagnosis of Herlyn-Werner-Wunderlich syndrome due to microperforation and pyocolpos in obstructed vaginal canal. J Pediatr Adolesc Gynecol. 2014;27(4):e79–81.
24. Siwatch S, Mehra R, Pandher DK. Rudimentary horn pregnancy: a 10 year experience and review of the literature. Arch Gynecol Obstet. 2013;287(4):687–95.
25. Khati NJ. The unicornuate uterus and its variants: a clinical presentation of imaging and associated findings and complications. J Ultrasound Med. 2012;213(31):319–31.
26. Hua M, Odibo AO, Longman RE, et al. Congenital uterine anomalies and adverse pregnancy outcomes. Am J Obstet Gynecol. 2011;205:558.
27. Fox NS, Roman AS, Strern EM, et al. Type of uterine anomaly and adverse pregnancy outcomes. J Matern Fetal Neonatal Med. 2014;27:949.
28. Fedele L, Bianchi S, Marchini M, et al. Ultrastructural aspects of endometrium in infertile women with septate uterus. Fertil Steril. 1996;65:750.
29. Reichman DE, Laufer MR. Congenital uterine anomalies affecting reproduction. Best Pract Res Clin Obstet Gynaecol. 2010;24(2):193–208.
30. Lavergne N, Aristizabal J, Zarka V, Erny R, Hedon B. Uterine anomalies and in vitro fertilization: what are the results? Eur J Obstet Gynecol Reprod Biol. 1996;68(1–2):29–34.
31. Raga F, Bauset C, Remohi J, Bonilla-Musoles F, Simon C, Pellicer A. Reproductive impact of congenital Müllerian anomalies. Hum Reprod. 1997;12(10):2277–81.
32. Chan YY et al. Reproductive outcomes in women with congenital uterine anomalies: a systematic review. Ultrasound Obstet Gynecol. 2011;38:371.
33. Pellerito JS et al. Diagnosis of uterine anomalies: relative accuracy of MR imaging, endovaginal sonography, and hysterosalpingography. Radiology. 1992;183(3):795–800.
34. Siam S, Soliman BS. Combined laparoscopy and hysteroscopy for the detection of female genital system anomalies results of 3,811 infertile women. J Reprod Med. 2014;59(11–12):542–6.
35. Siegel M. Female pelvis. In: Pediatric sonography. 4th ed. Philadelphia: Lippincott Williams & Wilkins; 2011. p. 509–53.
36. Garel L et al. US of the pediatric female pelvis: a clinical perspective. Radiographics. 2001;21(6):1393–407.
37. Langer JE et al. Imaging of the female pelvis through the life cycle. Radiographics. 2012;32(6):1575–97.
38. Thabet SM, Thabet AS. Role of new sono-imaging technique 'sonocolpography' in the diagnosis and treatment of the complete transverse vaginal septum and other allied conditions. J Obstet Gynaecol Res. 2002;28(2):80–5.
39. Son J, Taylor G. Transperineal ultrasonography. Pediatr Radiol. 2014;44(2):193–201.
40. Timor IE et al. Transrectal scanning: an alternative when transvaginal scanning is not feasible. Ultrasound Obstet Gynecol. 2003;21(5):473–9.
41. Chung T et al. Transrectal drainage of deep pelvic abscesses in children using a combined transrectal sonographic and fluoroscopic guidance. Pediatr Radiol. 1996;26(12):874–8.

42. Fedele L et al. Transrectal ultrasonography in the assessment of congenital vaginal canalization defects. Hum Reprod. 1999;14(2):359–62.
43. Riccabonna M. Three Dimensional Ultrasound based virtual cystoscopy of the pediatric urinary bladder: a preliminary report on feasibility and potential value. J Ultrasound Med. 2008;27(10):1453–9.
44. Bermejo C et al. Three-dimensional ultrasound in the diagnosis of Müllerian duct anomalies and concordance with magnetic resonance imaging. Ultrasound Obstet Gynecol. 2010;35(5):593–601.
45. Wu MH et al. Detection of congenital Mullerian duct anomalies using three-dimensional ultrasound. J Clin Ultrasound. 1997;25(9):487–92.
46. McCarville MB et al. Contrast-enhanced sonography of malignant pediatric abdominal and pelvic solid tumors: preliminary safety and feasibility data. Pediatr Radiol. 2012;42(7):824–33.
47. Yoo RE et al. A systematic approach to the magnetic resonance imaging-based differential diagnosis of congenital Müllerian duct anomalies and their mimics. Abdom Imaging. 2015;40(1):192–206.
48. Santos XM et al. The utility of ultrasound and magnetic resonance imaging versus surgery for the characterization of Müllerian anomalies in the pediatric and adolescent population. J Pediatr Adolesc Gynecol. 2012;25(3):181–4.
49. Lim K et al. Clinical application of 3D t@ weighted MRI in pelvic imaging. Abdom Imaging. 2014;39(5):1052–62.
50. Paltiel HJ, Phelps A. US of the pediatric female pelvis. Radiology. 2014;270(3):644–57.
51. Lermann J et al. Comparison of different diagnostic procedures for the staging of malformations associated with Mayer-Rokitansky-Küster-Hauser syndrome. Fertil Steril. 2011;96(1):156–9.
52. Oppelt PG. Malformations in a cohort of 284 women with Mayer-Rokitansky-Küster-Hauser syndrome (MRKH). Reprod Biol Endocrinol. 2012;10:57.
53. Creighton SM, Hall-Craggs M. Correlation or confusion: the need for accurate terminology when comparing magnetic resonance imaging and clinical assessment of congenital vaginal anomalies. J Pediatr Urol. 2010;8(2):177–80.
54. Junqueria BL et al. Mullerian duct anomalies and mimics in children and adolescents: correlative intraoperative assessment with clinical imaging. Radiographics. 2009;29(4):1085–103.
55. Calvo-Garcia MA et al. Fetal MRI clues to diagnose Cloacal Malformation. Pediatr Radiol. 2011;41(9):1117–28.
56. Acien P, Acien M, Sanchez-Ferrer M. Complex malformations of the female genital tract. New types and revision of classification. Hum Reprod. 2004;19:2377–84.
57. Bean EJ et al. Mayer-Rokitansky-Kuster-Hauser syndrome: sexuality, psychological effects, and quality of life. J Pediatr Adolesc Gynecol. 2009;22:339–46.
58. Brännström M et al. First clinical uterus transplantation trial: a six-month report. Fertil Steril. 2014;101(5):1228–36.

Part II

Vertical Anomalies

Imperforate Hymen

3

Julie Hakim and Jennifer E. Dietrich

Introduction

The development of the female reproductive tract is a complex series of events with numerous possibilities for abnormal development. Obstructive anomalies of the female reproductive tract can become apparent during childhood, puberty, or adolescence. In this chapter, the embryologic development of the female reproductive tract will be presented along with clinical descriptions of the imperforate hymen. Diagnosis and management including conservative and surgical options will be reviewed.

Incidence

Imperforate hymen is an uncommon obstructive anomaly of the female reproductive tract [1] but it is the most common cause of genital outflow obstruction in females [2]. Female reproductive tract abnormalities are generally encountered in 2–3 % of women [3], though incidence of imperforate hymen exists anywhere from 0.1 to 0.5 % of newborn girls [1].

J. Hakim, M.D. • J.E. Dietrich, M.D., M.Sc. (✉)
Baylor College of Medicine, 6651 Main St, Ste 1050,
Houston, TX 77030, USA
e-mail: jedietri@bcm.edu

Etiology

The exact function of the hymen is unknown. One proposed theory is that it acts [2] as a barrier to infections during the prepubertal period during which vaginal self-defense mechanisms have not yet fully developed.

Theories on the embryological genesis of uterovaginal anomalies are varied and have attempted to unify the various forms and combinations of uterovaginal anomalies seen together. Uniformly agreed upon, however, is that an imperforate hymen is the result of a failure of canalization [1] of the hymen during the perinatal period leading to an obstructed vaginal outflow tract. The uterus and vagina typically develop normally (Fig. 3.1). During embryogenesis, the paramesophrenic ducts fuse to form the uterovaginal primordium, which projects into the urogenital sinus and eventually induces the formation of the sinovaginal bulbs that fuse to form a solid vaginal plate. This plate later breaks down, forming the lumen of the vagina. The hymen is formed by invagination of the posterior wall of the urogenital sinus. The hymen usually ruptures during the perinatal period, leaving a thin mucous membrane at the entrance to the vagina of variable configuration, patent or non-patent. Regardless of patency, the normal hymen is described as thin and translucent during the prepubertal years, and pale pink with elasticity once puberty ensues.

© Springer International Publishing Switzerland 2016
S.M. Pfeifer (ed.), *Congenital Müllerian Anomalies*, DOI 10.1007/978-3-319-27231-3_3

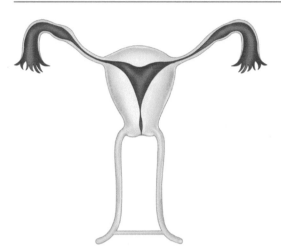

Fig. 3.1 Diagram showing imperforate hymen. Note the uterus, cervix, and vaginal structures are normal. The hymen at the introitus is occluded

A recent case report describing a patient with a uterovaginal septum and imperforate hymen highlights an alternate embryological theory of development given that the lower third of the vagina is thought to derive from the urogenital sinus. As such, the described association of a uterovaginal septum and imperforate hymen might alternately suggest an intertwined embryological derivation of these structures [4].

Another view is suggested by a study of patients with concurrent Rokitansky syndrome and hymenal variations [5]. Given that women without a hymen are also more likely to have renal tract anomalies, they postulate that in these patients the primary problem is with an underlying Wolffian duct or urogenital sinus defect rather than being primarily a Mullerian duct problem. Recently, a classification of vaginal malformations based on embryological, anatomical, and clinical criteria has been proposed [6]. They have identified six different moments in the embryogenesis phase in which the interruption of normal development of the vagina may lead to a malformation (Table 3.1) [6].

Unfortunately, the mode of inheritance of imperforate hymen is not yet known. Familial occurrences have been described, suggesting an autosomal dominant inheritance in some [7, 8]. Given the varied malformations associated with imperforate hymen, as well as case studies of nonsyndromic familial occurrences of imperforate hymen, the proposed mechanism of inheritance is thought to be by mutations in several genes, and mutations may differ from one family to another.

Diagnosis

The presentation of an imperforate hymen varies depending on the age of the patient. A recent study demonstrated a bimodal distribution of age

Table 3.1 Embryogenesis of vaginal malformations according to Ruggeri et al. [6]

Embryogenesis	Malformation	Type	Gestational age
Failure of development of mullerian ducts	MRKH	1A	6–8th week
	Isolated vaginal atresia	1B	8–9th week
Failure of development of urorectal septum	Cloaca	6	7th week
Failure of canalization of epithelial vaginal plate	Atresia	2	8th week
Failure of fusion of mullerian ducts	Duplication	5A	7th week
	Septum	5B	9th week
Defects in tuberculum of Muller	Atresia with proximal high UGS	3A	7–9th week
	Atresia with proximal low UGS	3B	13–18th week
Defect of resorption of mullerian septum	Transverse septum	4A	12–17th week
	Imperforate hymen	4B	20th week

Modified from Ruggeri G et al. [6]

at diagnosis [9] of imperforate hymen in a group of 23 girls where 43 % were diagnosed at <8 years of age, and 57 % were diagnosed at >8 years of age. They found that among the older girls, 100 % were symptomatic (abdominal pain and/or urinary symptoms; duration of symptoms: 1–120 days), whereas 90 % of cases in the younger group were detected incidentally.

In infants, maternal estrogen may stimulate uterovaginal secretions and cause hydrometrocolpos with a resultant bulging hymen called a mucocele [1]. Typically, this resolves spontaneously. However, occasionally, a large mucocele can result in functional urethral obstruction, necessitating intervention. With advances in ultrasonographic techniques and applicability, imperforate hymen can now be diagnosed by ultrasound in the prenatal period. For instance, if hematocolpometra is found on routine prenatal ultrasound, a more comprehensive ultrasound is performed for confirmation. Comprehensive prenatal ultrasound can also be used to distinguish between various obstructive uterovaginal anomalies [10]. In cases of equivocal prenatal ultrasound findings [11], or if anatomical relationships need further delineation, fetal MRI has become essential in comprehensive assessment of fetal genitourinary anomalies, settling prenatal diagnostic queries and assisting in surgical planning while reaching the accuracy of prenatal ultrasound.

The majority of girls with imperforate hymen are asymptomatic until adolescence [12]. The typical presentation is during puberty when the adolescent presents with lower abdominal pain in the setting of never having had a menstrual period (pre-menarche). Menstruation, however, has occurred with accumulation of menstrual blood in the obstructed vaginal canal leading to distention of the vagina, termed a hematocolpos. This mass can be very large measuring upwards of 10×15 cm and containing approximately 1 L of menstrual blood. This mass should be palpable and tender on abdominal exam. With further vaginal distention, the accumulated blood can back up into and distend the uterus termed hematometra. With continued pressure further retrograde menstruation occurs leading to the development of hematosalpinx, and development of endometriosis

Table 3.2 Common and uncommon presentations of imperforate hymen

Cyclic abdominal pain
Primary amenorrhea
Abdominal mass
Urinary retention
Constipation
Back pain
Hydronephrosis
Leg edema
Acute abdomen

Modified from Basaran M et al. [2]

and adhesions in the abdomen and pelvis. As the obstruction with imperforate hymen is at the opening of the vagina, and the vagina is distensible, it can accommodate a lot of blood before the development of hematometra of hematosalpinges occur. The extent of damage to the fallopian tubes and development of endometriosis is correlated with the delay in diagnosis.

The distended vagina and later hematometra/hematospinges cause pelvic or abdominal pain. This pain is usually cyclic reflecting menstruation and further accumulated blood in the obstructed cavity. However, as menstrual cycles in the first 2 years following menarche can be irregular, these pain symptoms may not be cyclic. As a result, they may be attributed to gastrointestinal causes and lead to delay in correct diagnosis. With time the pain may become continuous.

Approximately 58 % of patients may present with urinary hesitancy or dysuria in the presence of hematocolpos [2]. Patients may also present with (see Table 3.2) urinary retention [2] or low back pain [13], and changes in bowel habits. Others have suggested that imperforate hymen should be suspected in adolescent girls with symptoms of myofascial pain [13] who also have primary amenorrhea. Rare presentations include bilateral leg edema [12], venous dilatation in the inguinal region, renal tract obstruction caused by hydrometrocolpos, or ruptured hematosalpinx requiring laparoscopic salpingectomy.

Physical findings with imperforate hymen include a tender mass arising in the pelvis extending into the abdomen. Careful examination of the

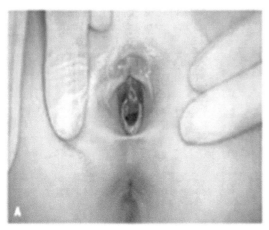
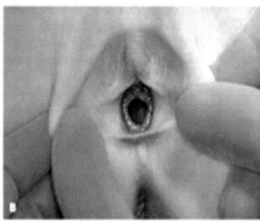

Fig. 3.2 Examination of the vulva, hymen, and anterior vagina by (**a**) gentle lateral retraction and (**b**) gentle gripping of the labia and pulling anteriorly (*Taken from Emans* *SJ, Laufer M. Pediatric and Adolescent Gynecology. 6th ed. Wolters-Kluwer: 2013* [14])

external genitalia can be performed using the "pull-down and towards you" traction maneuver for visualizing the entire vestibule and distal vagina in neonates and young children (Fig. 3.2). Examination of the vaginal opening reveals an obstruction at the introitus. No obvious hymenal ring is identified. With valsalva or abdominal pressure a distended hymen may be seen, typically with a bluish hue reflecting the collected menstrual blood above the hymen (Fig. 3.3a, b). A rectal exam may confirm the presence of a mass in the pelvis. However, some adolescents may not tolerate vaginal or rectal exam.

In the adolescent, diagnosis of imperforate hymen can be confirmed by ultrasound showing a distended vagina in the setting of amenorrhea and pelvic pain. As these anomalies are relatively rare, interpretation by an experienced radiologist is helpful. A recent study demonstrated that hematometrocolpos secondary to an imperforate hymen, as well as hydronephrosis, could be accurately diagnosed even in a pediatric emergency department setting using Point of Care Ultrasound (POCUS) [15] using POCUS views familiar to most PEM physicians. This point of care diagnosis had the potential to facilitate gynecological referral, PED disposition, definitive imaging in

the form of MRI, and surgical treatment. MRI may be helpful in confirming diagnosis, especially when differentiating an imperforate hymen from a low transverse vaginal septum as with an imperforate hymen, the lowest point of the distended vagina is typically lower than the pubic bone (Fig. 3.4a, b).

Associated Anomalies

Though most often an imperforate hymen is an isolated finding [7], it can be accompanied by malformations such as polydactyly, duplication of the ureter, ectopic ureter, urethral membrane, imperforate anus, hypoplastic or multicystic dysplastic kidney, and bifid clitoris [1]. Imperforate hymen has also been associated with Bardet-Biedl or McKusick-Kaufman syndromes. Bardet-Biedl syndrome is a heterogeneous group of autosomal recessive disorders characterized by retinal dystrophy or retinitis pigmentosa, post-axial polydactyly, obesity, renal dysfunction, and mental disturbances or mental retardation. McKusick-Kaufman syndrome [2, 12] is a rare autosomal recessive syndrome characterized by hydrometrocolpos, polydactyly, and congenital heart defects.

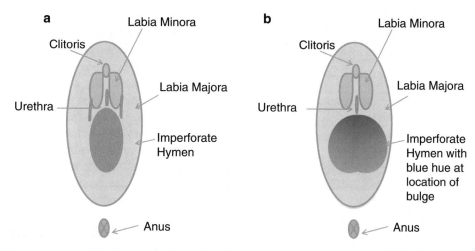

Fig. 3.3 (a) Diagram showing location of imperforate hymen. (b) Diagram showing location of the *Blue* hue seen with a thin imperforate hymen with valsalva

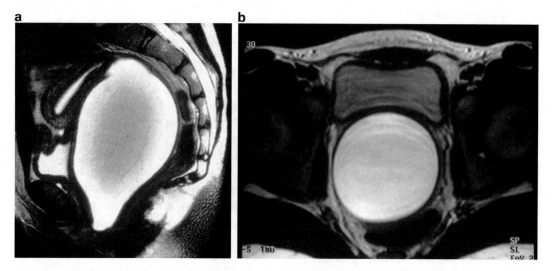

Fig. 3.4 (a) MRI T2 weighted image: Sagittal view of imperforate hymen. Note fluid within the obstructed vagina extends inferior to the pubic symphysis. Note there is no hematometra despite the large hematocolpos as the vagina is able to distend significantly (*Image provided by Samantha M. Pfeifer MD*). (b) MRI T2 weighted image: Transverse view of hematocolpos due to imperforate hymen. The diameter of the distended vagina is approximately 9 cm (*Image provided by Samantha M. Pfeifer MD*)

Differential Diagnoses

Imperforate hymen should be distinguished from a low transverse vaginal septum as the treatment of these two conditions is different. It is also important to differentiate imperforate hymen from vaginal agenesis prior to planning a surgical procedure. Imaging with ultrasound can be very helpful.

Other causes of vaginal obstruction that should be considered (Table 3.3) include obstructed hemivagina, vaginal agenesis, ambiguous genitalia, urethral prolapse, ectopic ureter, condyloma, rhabdomyosarcoma, labial adhesions, paraurethral cyst, and introital masses such as a Gartner duct cyst [17].

Table 3.3 Differential diagnoses

Imperforate hymen
1. Labial adhesions
2. Vaginal atresia
3. Vaginal agenesis
4. Low transverse vaginal septum
5. Ambiguous genitalia
6. Obstructed hemivagina
7. *Cystic mass at the introitus*
1. Imperforate hymen with hydrocolpos
2. Ectopic ureter with ureterocele
3. Urethral prolapse
4. Hymenal cyst
5. Hymenal skin tag
6. Periurethral cyst
7. Vaginal cyst
8. Rhabdomyosarcoma

Modified from The Ultrasound of Life www. fetalultrasound.com [16]

Treatment

Hymenectomy is widely accepted as the surgical treatment for [2] imperforate hymen. However, asymptomatic imperforate hymen may be managed conservatively, as in some cases the hymen may open spontaneously thereby obviating the need for surgical intervention [12, 18].

Standard treatment, however, is surgical hymenectomy with an incision in the shape of a "T," an "X," a plus sign, or cruciform shape with or without subsequent removal of the excess hymenal tissue [2]. If the excess hymenal tissue is not removed, this may increase the risk for re-occlusion. Cautery can be used for hemostasis. Care should be taken to avoid injury to the urethra and avoid resecting beyond the hymen as bleeding may be encountered [2]. An alternative technique has been described involving making an ovoid incision in the hymen, then placing a 16Fr Foley catheter through the incision, inflating the balloon, and placing estrogen cream on the hymenal area for 2 weeks [19]. Utilizing this technique the authors reported 63/65 patients had a patent vaginal hymen. Others suggest only topical estrogen cream postoperatively to promote wound healing and to decrease scar formation. The complications of a hymenectomy are bleeding, scarring, and stenosis of the vaginal

opening [20]. Virginity sparing hymenectomy procedure has been proposed which may be preferred in cultures and religious groups in which the integrity of the hymen is important [2]. This technique involves making a vertical incision, <1 cm in the hymen, then after drainage of the hematocolpos, the hymenal edges are then sutured obliquely to form a circular opening.

In cases of urinary retention due to hematometrocolpos, urethral catheterization is suggested as the first-line treatment [2]. In cases where this is unsuccessful, insertion of a suprapubic catheter can be performed. In patients with an infected hydrometrocolpos, urinary obstruction and severe septicemia who are not candidates for general anesthesia, percutaneous drainage through the lower abdominal wall with mild sedation as an effective means of relieving the obstruction, with surgical intervention once the individual's general condition improves.

For those individuals diagnosed with an asymptomatic imperforate hymen prior to puberty, the timing of hymenectomy has traditionally been around the time of puberty. However, there remains some debate given patients with imperforate hymen may be at higher risk of endometriosis and vaginal adenosis [13]. Literature supporting these theories is limited. Physicians must weigh the risks of anesthesia, smaller anatomy, and potentially poorer tissue healing for young children against the potential adverse outcomes resulting from postponed correction.

Finally, physicians should be aware that surgical management of imperforate hymen might have different connotations and/or sociocultural consequences for patients in different cultures and religious groups. As such, discussions around surgical recommendations should be undertaken with care, balancing health advocacy and cultural sensitivity.

Impact on Fertility and Reproduction

Mechanism for infertility associated with imperforate hymen relates to tubal damage and scarring due to endometriosis as a result of forced retrograde menstruation in the setting of vaginal obstruction. As discussed above, the vagina is distensible and can accommodate a significant amount of menstrual blood before retrograde menstruation and endometriosis occurs. One study evaluating fertility in patients who had an imperforate hymen diagnosed at puberty found that of the 22 patients treated, 86 % conceived suggesting little if any affect on fertility [21]. However, the longer the delay in diagnosis the more upper tract damage may occur.

Conclusion

Imperforate hymen is an uncommon obstructive anomaly of the female reproductive tract. The presentation of an imperforate hymen varies depending on the age of the patient. Signs and symptoms can range from asymptomatic, to a mucocele visible in a neonate, to intermittent pelvic or abdominal pain that is usually cyclic in the adolescent who is premenarcheal. Other symptoms may include urinary retention or constipation. The inheritance pattern of imperforate hymen is still unclear, though it is largely an isolated finding. Diagnosis can be confirmed by ultrasound, typically in the setting of pelvic or abdominal pain in a premenarcheal girl. We highlight the importance of a thorough history and physical exam including Tanner staging to prevent delays in diagnosis. Management by hymenectomy is the standard of care with usually excellent results.

References

1. Yun-Hsuen L, Soon Pheng N, Jamil M. Imperforate hymen: report of an unusual familial occurrence. J Obstet Gynaecol. 2003;29(6):399–401.
2. Basaran M, Usal D, Aydemir C. Hymen sparing surgery for imperforate hymen: case reports and review of literature. J Pediatr Adolesc Gynecol. 2009;22: e61–4.
3. Deligeoroglou E, Deliveliotou A, Makrakis E, Creatsas G. Concurrent imperforate hymen, transverse vaginal septum, and unicornuate uterus: a case report. J Pediatr Surg. 2007;42:1446–8.
4. Fedele L, Frontino G, Motta F, Restelli E. A uterovaginal septum and imperforate hymen with a double

pyocolpos. Hum Reprod. 2012;27(6):1637–9. doi:10.1093/humrep/des084.
5. Kimberley N, Hutson JM, Southwell BR, Grover SR. Vaginal agenesis, the hymen, and associated anomalies. J Pediatr Adolesc Gynecol. 2012;25(1):54–8. doi:10.1016/j.jpag.2011.08.003.
6. Ruggeri G, Gargano T, Antonellini C, Carlini V, et al. Vaginal malformations: a proposed classification based on embryological, anatomical and clinical criteria and their surgical management (an analysis of 167 cases). Pediatr Surg Int. 2012;28:797–803.
7. Stelling JR, Gray MR, Davis AJ, Cowan JM, Reindollar RH. Dominant transmission of imperforate hymen. Fertil Steril. 2000;74:1241–4.
8. Usta IM, Awwad JT, Makarem MM, Karam KS. Imperforate hymen: report of an unusual familial occurrence. Obstet Gynecol. 1993;82:655–6.
9. Posner J, Spandorfer P. Early Detection of Imperforate Hymen Prevents Morbidity from Delays in Diagnosis. Pediatrics. 2005;115(4):10008–12.
10. Bhargava P, Dighe M. Prenatal US diagnosis of congenital imperforate hymen. Pediatr Radiol. 2009; 39:1014. doi:10.1007/s00247.
11. Capito C, Belarbi N, Jaouen A, Leger J, Carel JC, Oury JF, Sebag G, El-Ghoneimi A. Prenatal pelvic MRI: additional clues for assessment of urogenital obstructive anomalies. J Pediatr Urol. 2014;10:162e–166.
12. Nagai K, Murakami Y, Nagatani K, Nakahashi N, et al. Life-threatening acute renal failure due to imperforate hymen in an infant. Pediatr Int. 2012;54(2):280–2. doi:10.1111/j/1442-200X.2011.03422.x.
13. Domany E, Gilad O, Shwarz M, Vulfsons S, Zion GB. Imperforate hymen presenting as chronic low back pain. Pediatrics. 2013;132, e768. doi:10.1542/peds. 2012-1040.
14. Emans SJ, Laufer M. Pediatric and adolescent gynecology. 6th ed. Philadelphia: Wolters-Kluwer; 2013.
15. Fischer JW, Kwan CW. Emergency point-of-care ultrasound diagnosis of hematocolpometra and imperforate hymen in the pediatric emergency department. Pediatr Emerg Care. 2014;30(2):128–30.
16. The Ultrasound of Life. http://www.fetalultrasound. com. Accessed 11 Nov 2014.
17. Wolfson A, Hendey GW, Ling LJ, Rosen C, Schaider J, Sharieff G. Harwood-Nuss' clinical practice of emergency medicine. 5th ed. Philadelphia: Wolters; 2009.
18. Kahn R, Duncan B, Bowes W. Spontaneous opening of congenital imperforate hymen. J Pediatr. 1975;87: 768–9.
19. Acar A, Balci O, Karatayli R, Capar M, Colakoglu MC. The treatment of 65 women with imperforate hymen by a central incision and application of Foley catheter. BJOG. 2007;114(11):1376–9.
20. Lardenoije C, Aardenburg R, Mertens H. Imperforate hymen: a cause of abdominal pain in female adolescents. BMJ Case Rep. 2009;2009.
21. Rock JA, Zacur HA, Dlugi AM, Jones HW, TeLinde RW. Pregnancy success following surgical correction of imperforate hymen and complete transverse vaginal septum. Obstet Gynecol. 1982;59:448.

Transverse Vaginal Septum

4

Veronica I. Alaniz and Elisabeth H. Quint

Introduction and Incidence

Transverse vaginal septa are a rare type of mullerian anomaly that results from failed fusion or canalization of the vaginal plate and the caudal end of the mullerian ducts, leading to a complete or partial blockage of the vaginal canal. The exact incidence is not known and estimates ranging between 1:21,000 [1] and 1:84,000 [2] are based on limited data. Transverse vaginal septa are unlikely to be associated with other mullerian anomalies; however, there are case reports of transverse septa with a septate uterus [3], unicornuate uterus, and hymenal abnormalities [4–6]. Concurrent renal anomalies, as seen with other mullerian anomalies, occasionally occur with transverse vaginal septa [7].

There is no accepted classification system for congenital vaginal anomalies among the American and European gynecologic societies. The American Society for Reproductive Medicine (ASRM) classification for mullerian anomalies only includes vaginal agenesis and hypoplasia (Type 1A), however does allow for the description of associated vaginal anomalies [8]. The European Society of Human Reproduction and Embryology (ESHRE) and the European Society for Gynaecological Endoscopy (ESGE) include transverse vaginal septa, but only as a subclass (V3) in their classification system for mullerian anomalies [9]. There have been several proposed classification systems for vaginal anomalies, including the VCUAM classification and an embryological-clinical based system [10–12]. See Chap. 1 for more details.

Transverse vaginal septa have a variety of characteristics including position in the vagina, thickness, and presence of perforations. Position is generally described as low, mid, or high (Figs. 4.1 and 4.2), though there is no accepted system for classifying the location and a variety of measurements are used in the literature. In a recent observational study, the largest to date, septal location was described as the distance measured in clinic or during an exam under anesthesia between the vaginal introitus and the distal end of the septum [13]. Septa were classified as low if less than 3 cm, mid position if between 3 and 6 cm, and high if greater than 6 cm from the introitus. In this study, the most common location was low (72 %), followed by mid position (22 %), and high (6 %) [13]. In a review of the literature from 1966 to 1997, location of the septum was reported in 67 patients and described as low (distal 1–3 cm) in 20 %, mid (4–5 cm) in 33 %, and high (>6 cm) in 47 % of patients [14].

V.I. Alaniz, M.D., M.P.H. • E.H. Quint, M.D. (✉)
Department of Obstetrics and Gynecology, University of Michigan Health System, 1500 E Medical Center Drive, SPC 5276, Ann Arbor, MI 48109, USA
e-mail: Alaniz@med.umich.edu;
Equint@med.umich.edu

© Springer International Publishing Switzerland 2016
S.M. Pfeifer (ed.), *Congenital Müllerian Anomalies*, DOI 10.1007/978-3-319-27231-3_4

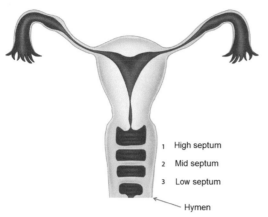

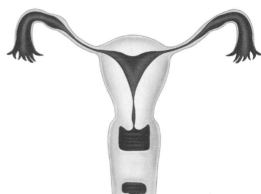

Fig. 4.1 Location of transverse vaginal septum

Fig. 4.3 Thick transverse vaginal septum (distal vaginal agenesis)

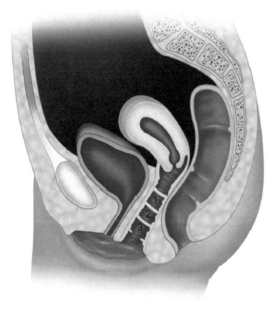

Fig. 4.2 Diagram showing location of High (1), Mid (2), and Low (1) transverse vaginal Septum in pelvis

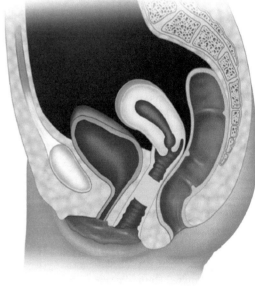

Fig. 4.4 Diagram showing location of thick transverse vaginal septum in pelvis

The thickness of septum is the most important characteristic in terms of surgical planning. Septa are considered thin if less than 1 cm and thick if greater than 1 cm [15] (Figs. 4.3 and 4.4). Fortunately, most septa are less than 1 cm in thickness [8, 16]; however, in about 15 % of cases a several centimeter thick septum is present and can be considered partial vaginal agenesis or atresia [17]. In general, thicker septa occur higher in the vagina [18]. Most (61–65 %) transverse septa are imperforate [13, 14]. When a perforation is

present, it is usually small and centrally located, but eccentric, bilateral, and multiple perforations have also been described [14] (Fig. 4.5).

Etiology

Embryologic development of the vagina begins around 9 weeks gestation, when the distal mullerian ducts fuse to form the uterovaginal canal. The mullerian ducts contribute to the upper

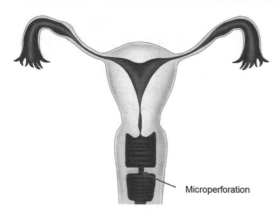

Microperforation

Fig. 4.5 Transverse vaginal septum with microperforation

portion of the vagina, whereas the lower portion arises from the urogenital sinus. At 12 weeks the sinovaginal bulbs develop as two solid evaginations from the mullerian tubercle on the urogenital sinus. The sinovaginal bulbs grow into the uterovaginal canal and develop a solid vaginal plate of stratified squamous epithelium [8]. The solid vaginal plate proliferates toward the cephalad direction, replacing the original mullerian epithelium with squamous epithelium [2]. It then cannulates which is complete by 5 months gestation. The hymen, which typically perforates at birth, originates from the caudal end of the sinovaginal bulbs [8].

The embryologic etiology of transverse vaginal septa is controversial and cannot be solely explained by failed fusion of the urogenital sinus and mullerian ducts; this would lead to formation of transverse septa in the lower one-third of the vagina only, while in fact, septa can be located at many different levels in the vagina (Figs. 4.1 and 4.2). It is hypothesized that the squamous epithelium that invaginates from the vaginal plate can leave behind vestigial shreds during canalization causing septa to form at different locations in the vagina [14, 19].

Isolated vaginal anomalies likely have a polygenic or multifactorial inheritance pattern. McKusick-Kaufman Syndrome (MKS) is an autosomal recessive condition caused by mutations in the *MKKS* gene. In females with MKS, transverse vaginal septa as well as vaginal agenesis or imperforate hymen are found in association with polydactyly and congenital cardiac defects [20, 21].

Differential Diagnosis

When a patient presents with an obstructive vaginal anomaly, clinicians should consider imperforate hymen, transverse vaginal septum, cervical agenesis, and vaginal atresia in the differential diagnosis. An imperforate hymen, the most common obstructive anomaly, can easily be diagnosed with visualization. Though the presence of a patent hymen can usually be confirmed at an early age on genital examination, an imperforate hymen is often not recognized until after menarche. Typically, a membranous bulge is seen at the introitus and the hymen presents as a solid plate. The mass increases with a valsalva maneuver and can be confirmed on rectal examination with a low lying bulge, extending almost to the rectal orifice [8, 16, 17]. See Chap. 3 for more details.

Cervical agenesis, congenital absence of the cervix and/or upper vagina, is a rare anomaly that is important to diagnosis correctly. Absence of a cervix on MRI is the feature that distinguishes this anomaly from other obstructive anomalies [8]. Details on the presentation and management are discussed in Chap. 5. Vaginal atresia, or agenesis of the lower vagina, occurs when the lower vagina fails to develop from the urogenital sinus and is instead replaced by fibrous tissue. This leads to an obstructed upper vagina and clinically presents like an imperforate transverse septum. Examination of the external genitalia reveals a normal hymen, vaginal dimple and on rectal exam a high bulge is palpated from a blood filled upper vagina [8, 16]. Adolescents with complete vaginal agenesis (MRKH) who have uterine remnants with functioning endometrium can also present with obstructive symptoms [16]. This should be considered in patients with a vaginal dimple who do not have a palpable bulge on rectal exam. Most of these anomalies can be diagnosed correctly with a proper physical exam, including a rectal exam, and appropriate imaging.

Patients with a perforated transverse vaginal septum have a more variable presentation which does not include amenorrhea. The differential diagnosis includes all conditions and anomalies that preclude visualization of the cervix, inability to place tampons, dyspareunia, or inability to have intercourse.

Diagnosis

Presentation

A transverse vaginal septum can be diagnosed during infancy, childhood, adolescence, or adulthood. The symptoms vary and are dependent on whether the septum is imperforate or perforate. A complete vaginal transverse septum leads to obstruction of the outflow tract, which presents as mucocolpos during infancy or hematocolpos shortly after menarche. Incomplete vaginal septa are usually diagnosed at a later age with a more variable presentation.

- *Complete (imperforate) transverse vaginal septum*: The most common presentation, usually occurring 2–3 years after thelarche, is primary amenorrhea with worsening cyclic pelvic pain. Hematocolpos and sometimes hematometra develops from accumulated menstrual blood which in extreme cases may present as an abdominopelvic mass. Patients complain of moderate to severe pain located in the abdomen, pelvis, or back. Pain can be significant enough to cause nausea and vomiting as well as school absences and frequent visits to the pediatrician or emergency department [17]. Adolescents with a high septum tend to present earlier because the upper vagina and uterus distend quickly with blood, causing severe pain [16]. In a series of 46 patients with transverse vaginal septa, 61 % were imperforate, diagnosed at a mean age of 14.3 years with primary amenorrhea and pain due to obstructed menstruation. One patient presented with cyclical hematuria due to a vagino-vesical fistula [13]. Though rare, obstructions can develop in the neonatal period as a result of increased vaginal and cervical secretions from exposure to maternal estrogen. In infants, a large hydrometrocolpos can cause symptoms related to compression of the ureters, rectum, and vena cava, which can be life threatening from resulting cardiorespiratory failure [22, 23].
- *Incomplete (perforate) transverse vaginal septum*: Patients with a perforate septum usually have a normal menarche and are more likely to present in late adolescence or young adulthood with complaints of difficulty inserting tampons, dyspareunia, dysmenorrhea, or infertility. Pyocolpos from an ascending infection, abnormal discharge, or abnormal bleeding can also occur in the setting of a partial obstruction, but is more uncommon [13, 14, 24]. The reported mean age of diagnosis is 24 years [13].

Physical Examination

- *Complete (imperforate) transverse vaginal septum*: Visualization of the external genitalia should reveal a normal open hymenal ring, which helps to distinguish a transverse septum from an imperforate hymen. In the young adolescent, a small and lubricated Q-tip can sometimes be used to assess the distance from the hymen to the obstruction. The physician should avoid touching the hymen, which is especially sensitive and causes pain in many young patients [17]. For those that can tolerate a speculum or digital exam, the vagina appears short and is often described as a "blind pouch." If the septum is thin, a bulge might be palpated or seen in the vagina from the distended upper vagina. A rectal exam, which is often better tolerated than a vaginal exam, can help delineate the lower edge of the septum by measuring the distance from the rectal opening to the bottom of the vaginal bulge (Fig. 4.6). If the obstruction is high or longstanding, an abdominal mass due to a distended vagina and uterus can be palpated [16, 24, 25].
- *Incomplete (imperforate) transverse vaginal septum*: Since these patients usually present at a later age, a pelvic exam with a speculum is generally tolerated. The external genitalia and hymen are normal and upon insertion of the speculum a short vagina is noted and no cervix is seen; the length of the lower vagina is dependent on the location of the septum. The septal perforation opening can usually be identified by inspection or gentle probing with a Q-tip. If no opening is seen, the patient should be reexamined during her menses, as blood can aid in identifying a microperforation (Figs. 4.7 and 4.8).

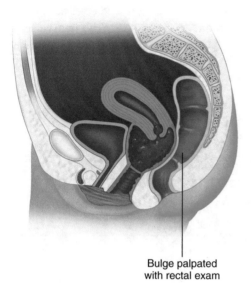

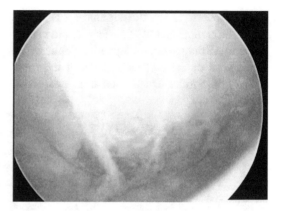

Fig. 4.8 View of cervix via hysteroscope passed through microperforation in transverse vaginal septum (*image provided by Samantha M. Pfeifer M.D.*)

Bulge palpated
with rectal exam

Fig. 4.6 Diagram of transverse vaginal septum with distended upper vagina that may be palpated on rectal exam

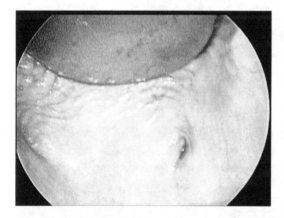

Fig. 4.7 Transverse vaginal septum microperforation (*image provided by Samantha M. Pfeifer M.D.*)

Laboratory Studies Laboratory studies do not aid in the diagnosis of a transverse vaginal septum. If tumor markers are drawn as part of the evaluation of the abdominopelvic mass, then CA 125 and/or CA 19-9 may be elevated [26].

Imaging A pelvic ultrasound is typically the first line imaging modality for gynecological structures but is limited in evaluating complex anatomy. Three-dimensional (3D) ultrasound has been found useful in diagnosing uterine malformations;

however, studies on the efficacy of 3D ultrasound in diagnosing vaginal anomalies are limited [27]. MRI is highly specific and sensitive for identifying mullerian tract anomalies, while also providing information on associated genitourinary abnormalities. Since an adequate MRI requires the patient to lie still for a period of time, general anesthesia or sedation may be necessary in young girls or anxious adolescents. Though MRI is more expensive than Computed Tomography (CT) scan, it provides high resolution and detailed images of the anatomy without exposure to radiation [28].

In general T2 weighted sequences are most helpful in evaluating internal pelvic structures. The zonal anatomy of the uterus, cervix, and vagina are delineated with varying signal intensities; the vagina has bright mucosa with a darker submucosa. T1 weighted sequences do not depict zonal anatomy but are helpful in delineating obstructed blood flow, which appears as a bright signal [29].

The literature supports the use of MRI as the gold standard for evaluation of upper mullerian tract anomalies; however, MRI evaluation of the vagina is more challenging [30]. In a retrospective review of 44 patients with a variety of congenital anomalies of the genitourinary tract, 30 of which had abnormal vaginal anatomy including vaginal agenesis, there was a 6.8 % discordance between clinical and imaging findings on the first review. This study emphasizes the importance of a multidisciplinary discussion about the clinical and MRI findings to aid in final and correct diagnosis of vaginal anomalies. The caudal end of the urethra, located at the same level of the hymen, can be used as an anatomical marker for the introitus when measuring vaginal length on MRI (Fig. 4.9). With transverse vaginal septum, there should be clear identification of the cervical canal to differentiate from cervical agenesis (Fig. 4.10).

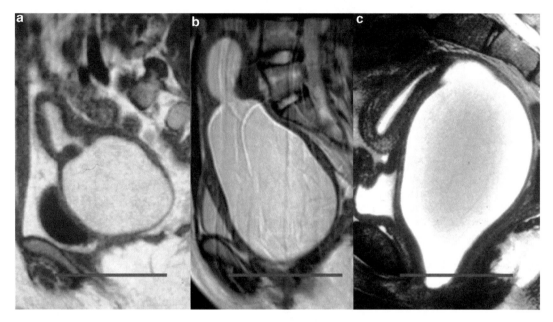

Fig. 4.9 (**a**, **b**) MRI sagittal T2 weighted images of transverse vaginal septum demonstrating clear cervix and distended upper vagina superior to symphysis. (**c**) MRI image of imperforate hymen (*image provided by Samantha M. Pfeifer M.D.*)

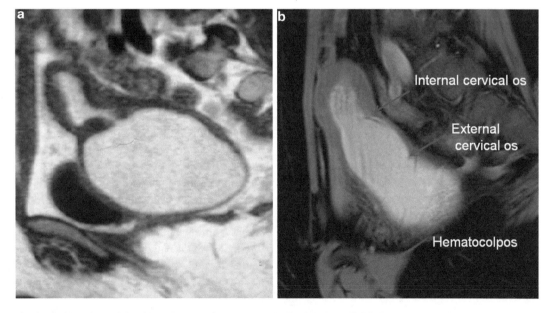

Fig. 4.10 MRI, T2 weighted image, view of cervix. (**a**) clear cervical canal (**b**) distended uterus, cervix, and vagina, making identification of cervix more difficult (*image provided by Samantha M. Pfeifer M.D.*)

Another technique for marking the introitus on MRI is placement of external oil beads at the level of the hymen prior to imaging [31]. Surgilube, which acts as a contrast agent, can be placed in the vagina to help delineate complex vaginal anomalies, or when the vaginal walls are collapsed, as is the case with a perforate transverse vaginal septum [32]. While some report the use of tampons as helpful in highlighting the vagina, others report that tampons obscure vaginal wall anatomy in MRI [31, 33].

- *Complete (imperforate) transverse vaginal septum*: The initial diagnosis of obstruction is often made with ultrasound by identifying a cystic mass in the vagina and/or a uterus distended with blood products. This provides the diagnosis, but does not give enough detail of the anatomy, location, and thickness of the septum. Because surgical technique changes based on the location and thickness of the septum, attempts should be made to fully characterize the septum preoperatively by MRI.
- *Incomplete (perforate) transverse vaginal septum*. Imaging for the thickness of the perforate transverse septum is more challenging, as the anatomy is harder to characterize with collapsed vaginal walls. In these cases, MRI can be considered using the above-described techniques.

Treatment

The goals of treatment are to relieve the obstruction if present and restore anatomy so that the vagina can function for menstrual outflow and coitus. Anomalies that are obstructive require immediate attention to resolve symptoms, whereas surgical resection of a perforate septum is elective. Hormonal suppression of menses with delay in surgery can be considered while the appropriate testing is performed. The patients' age, developmental level, and ability to perform postoperative dilation factors into the decision making and in certain cases, longer delays to surgery may be necessary.

The location and especially the thickness of septum are important characteristics in terms of surgical planning. In general, low and thin septa are less complicated, easier to resect, and require less postoperative care.

The outer surface of a transverse septum resembles normal vaginal mucosa and histologically is stratified squamous epithelium. The histopathology of the obstructed side of the septum varies, but in general the upper vagina is lined with glandular columnar epithelium and typically appears more erythematous. After resection of the septum, the upper vagina will undergo a metaplastic process and transform into squamous epithelium [23, 24].

Primary Resection and Anastomosis

Treatment of a thin septum is typically straightforward and requires resection of the septum followed by end-to-end anastomosis of the upper and lower vaginal mucosa. After placement of a catheter to keep the bladder drained, the initial incision should be made in the center of the septum, with an assistant using abdominal pressure to create or increase a bulge. If a bulge is not easily appreciated, then transabdominal ultrasound can be used to help establish a connection to the upper vagina. A spinal needle, under ultrasound guidance can be used to find the obstructed space, a wire is then placed in the obstructed area and sequential dilation of the septum over the wire can subsequently be performed. The incision is then stretched and obstructed blood evacuated. The inner vaginal walls and cervix should be palpated before resecting the residual septum. Resection of the septum in its entirety decreases the risk of stenosis and re-obstruction [34]. If the septum is high in the vagina, a Foley catheter can be placed through the initial incision and behind the septum. The catheter balloon is then filled with saline and pulled against the septum, which allows for easier resection of the septum [35].

The upper and lower vagina should be re-approximated with a delayed absorbable suture (such as 3-0 polysorb) in an interrupted fashion to minimize postoperative constriction [34]. Anastomosis tends to be easier when the upper vagina is distended with menstrual blood, by expanding the upper vaginal walls and providing more tissue for surgery [15].

Resection of thick septa is associated with increased risk of injury to nearby structures including bowel, bladder, and cervix. Surgical correction of a thick septum is more complicated and often requires undermining and mobilization of the upper vagina to aid in re-anastomosis without tension on the suture line (pull through procedure). The initial incision into a thick septum can be challenging; however, there are several techniques that can aid in establishing the connection between the upper and lower vagina. Interventional radiology can be consulted to place a catheter through the septum into the distended upper vagina under ultrasound guidance. The septum is then carefully resected around the catheter, paying special attention to orientation and nearby structures [34]. Another option is utilizing a transabdominal or laparoscopic approach to resect a high septum, an approach that works better when the upper vagina has been dilated with blood products. The push through technique is another option for thick transverse septa. After creating a bladder flap, the upper vagina is opened (with care taken not to enter through the potentially dilated and thinned cervix) and the obstructed blood is removed. A blunt object, such as a sterile marble, is placed in the upper vagina. Tension from the sterile object allows for better visualization and easier resection of the septum vaginally [35]. Alternatively, a sound can be passed through the fundus and into the upper vagina in an effort to help identify the vaginal septum from below [25].

A Z-plasty incision may help prevent circumferential scarring by changing the axis of the suture line so that scar contracts in a longitudinal fashion rather than a transverse fashion. The first step in performing a Z-plasty is making two oblique and crossed incisions over the lower edge of the vaginal septum. Using oblique incisions minimizes risk of injury to the bladder and rectum. The vaginal tissue is then undermined, creating four triangular shaped mucosal flaps of vagina, which can be tagged with suture to help with orientation and traction. The connective tissue in the septum should then be sharply dissected off the vaginal wall and removed. The inner vaginal lining of the septum is then incised with two crossed incisions, rotated 45° from the outer incisions. The flaps are undermined until mobilized enough for anastomosis. The apex of each flap is joined to the basal intersection of the two opposite flaps to form a continuous Z-plasty. This technique (Garica Z-plasty with Grunberger modification) was successfully performed on a series of 13 patients with both obstructed and nonobstructed transverse vaginal septa. In this series, the thickness of septa ranged from 2 to 3.5 cm and patients were followed for a mean of 6.3 years postoperatively. Vaginal lengths ranged from 9 to 12 cm and there were no patients with signs of vaginal contracture. Eight of the patients were known to eventually have a vaginal delivery [7].

Resection of a thick septum has the potential to leave a gap between the distal and proximal vagina. If native vaginal tissue cannot be mobilized enough to cover the resected area, other tissue is needed to create a patent vaginal canal. Options for closing this gap include use of bowel, skin, or buccal mucosal grafts. The disadvantages of skin grafting include risk of postoperative vaginal stenosis and scarring at the graft site [13]. Bowel interposition, a much larger operation, is associated with less stenosis and usually does not require postoperative dilation; however, patients do report copious vaginal discharge [24]. Vaginoplasty with buccal mucosa offers many advantages over skin grafting and bowel interposition; it eliminates the need for abdominal surgery, provides moist pliable mucosa without hair, and has a hidden donor site [36, 37]. Postoperative mouth pain is usually short and well tolerated. Vaginal tissue engineering is a promising option for vaginal reconstruction and has been used successfully in small numbers of patients with MRKH [38]. Postoperative hospital admission should be considered if a graft is used, requiring immobilization and Foley catheter use.

The risk of postoperative scarring and stenosis of the surgical area is higher with the thick septa and may require repeat surgery [13]. Postoperative dilation is recommended for most septal resections, however given the rarity of these anomalies, there is minimal outcome data and little information about the best method for postoperative dilation. In the original description by Rock in Telinde's Gynecology, a hollow vaginal mold was used that allowed outflow of menstrual blood. Typically silicone dilators or vaginal molds made of soft foam and covered with a latex condom are used. If the dilator is small enough to fit above the levator ani muscles, it will usually stay in the vagina without any additional support [23]. Custom made molds (10.5 cm in length with a diameter of 2.6 cm) with harness-like belts to keep the dilator in place have been described [39]. Alternatively, the use of tight spandex shorts can be helpful in keeping firm dilators in the vagina for prolonged periods of time. Postoperatively, after resolution of hematometra, the patient should wear a vaginal stent or dilator continuously for around 2 months to prevent stenosis or re-obstruction. Patients should be advised that they may need to remove the dilator for bowel movements or urination. If the surgical site is healing well and there are no complications, dilator use can be decreased to nighttime only for several more months and then intermittent until sexual activity is started [34]. Frequent vaginal examination will help to individualize dilator use.

Short-term and long-term complications of vaginal septum resection include bladder, bowel, and cervical injuries during surgery, infection, and vaginal stenosis or re-obstruction. A bladder catheter should be placed during surgery and cystouretheroscopy considered to rule out injury to the bladder. Frequent rectal exams during the surgery can be used to maintain orientation and prevent rectal injury. Efforts should be made to identify the dilated ectocervix on preoperative MRI. A dilated cervix can resemble vaginal wall, therefore caution should be used when resecting a septum located near the cervix. If it is unclear where vagina ends and cervix begins, a biopsy of the tissue can be taken for frozen section.

In William's study of 46 patients with transverse vaginal septa, 15 patients (33 %) had a high septum that was managed with an abdominoperineal approach. Short-term complications after surgery occurred in 27 % of those patients and included vessel injury, wound infection, pyometra, and pneumonia. Five patients (33 %) had recurrent obstructions that were treated with hysterectomy in two patients and repeat vaginal surgery in three patients. One patient had vaginal stenosis that was treated with dilation. Of the 27 patients (59 %) who underwent a vaginal approach, there were no short-term complications and two cases of vaginal stenosis (7 %) that were treated with dilation. Fourteen percent of patients in this study had already undergone one surgical procedure and were having a second surgery for re-obstruction [13].

Drainage and Suppression of Menstruation

The patient's psychological maturity and age should be considered when exploring surgical options for a transverse vaginal septum. If there are concerns that the patient cannot comply with postoperative dilation, then a delayed repair can be considered. Hormonal suppression of menses with or without drainage of the hematocolpos allows for delayed surgery and improved compliance with postoperative dilation in select patients. Decompression of hematocolpos has been described but carries a potential risk of ascending infection [16]. Hurst and Rock have reported ultrasound guided aspiration as a method to relieve acute pain associated with hematocolpos. The three patients in this report received broad spectrum prophylactic antibiotics with one postoperative infection [40]. In a review of patients at Royal Hospital for Women, three patients with lower vaginal agenesis had an attempted vaginal drainage of hematocolpos prior to referral, all of which became infected [41]. Laparoscopic drainage of hematocolpos has also been described as an approach in managing acute symptoms, which theoretically carries a lower risk of infection, because the upper vaginal cavity remains relatively sterile [42]. Hematocolpos acts as a natural tissue expander; therefore, once decompressed, the septum may become thicker and more difficult to treat.

Delayed Anastomosis

If diagnosed early and a symptomatic obstruction has not yet developed, menstrual suppression with continuous oral contraceptive pills, depot medroxyprogesterone acetate, or GnRH agonists followed by delayed anastomosis can be considered [34]. Delay allows for a period of preoperative dilation of the lower vagina in patients with a thick septum, which will increase the amount of native vaginal tissue available for re-anastomosis and may alleviate the need for grafts [40, 43].

Expectant management should be considered in the asymptomatic young girl who is diagnosed with a transverse septum before menarche. Delaying surgery until after puberty allows gradual development of hematocolpos, which can flatten the septum. Surgery is then less complicated with a thin septum and estrogenized epithelium. This approach was described in a case report and after 9 months of expectant management, a thick transverse septum decreased from 26 mm in thickness to 8 mm [44].

Infants with mucocolpos due to a transverse vaginal septum can usually be managed expectantly unless the obstruction is causing compression of nearby structures. In the rare circumstance, when the fluid collection is large enough to compress the ureters, rectum, or vena cava, the septum is life threatening and requires urgent surgical management [45]. Infants undergoing early surgery may require repeat surgery and should be followed closely through puberty [23].

Impact on Fertility and Reproduction

Patients with obstructing transverse septa can develop endometriosis from retrograde menstruation. In a study by Rock et al., seven patients with a transverse septum undergoing surgical correction had a concurrent laparotomy, diagnosing endometriosis in 86 % of those cases. The risk of endometriosis increases with imperforate septa that are located higher in the vagina [46]. Williams et al. report a 42 % incidence of endometriosis among low septa, 50 % among mid septa, and 100 % among high septa. The risk of tubal dysfunction increases if the obstruction results in hematosalpinx. Sexual activity and subsequent fertility can also be affected by psychosocial stressors associated with diagnosis and treatment, vaginal stenosis, dyspareunia, and re-obstruction.

Limited reproductive outcome data is available. Williams et al. reported data on seven patients who attempted pregnancy in their series of 46; they all achieved pregnancy with three vaginal deliveries, three cesarean deliveries, and one early termination. This limited reproductive outcome data may be the result of a young patient population and/or response bias in returning mailed questionnaires [13]. Rock et al. report increased rates of infertility and endometriosis among obstructive transverse septa compared to imperforate hymens. Among 19 patients who attempted pregnancy after surgical correction of a transverse septum, 9 conceived (47 %) and 7 had live births (36 %) [46].

There are reports of asymptomatic perforated transverse septa discovered in pregnancy. Proposed management for these cases includes resection of the septum before labor, prophylactic cesarean delivery, and expectant management allowing for spontaneous delivery with option to incise the septum as needed during the second stage of labor. Many argue that prophylactic cesarean delivery is indicated when a transverse septum is diagnosed in pregnancy to avoid vaginal laceration, scarring, and labor obstruction [47]. Others have challenged the need for prophylactic cesarean delivery by reporting two patients who had successful vaginal deliveries after incision of the septa in active labor. Though challenging during labor, because cervical dilatation cannot easily be assessed and internal monitors cannot be used, expectant management may be an option for patients with thin, perforate septa [48].

References

1. Lodi A. Contribuo clinic statistic sulle malformazione all vagina osservate nella. Clinca Obstetricia e Gynecoligia di Mmilano dal 1906–1950. Ann Ostet Ginecol. 1951;73:1246–51.

2. Wenof M, Reynaih JV, Novendstern J, Castadot MJ. Transverse vaginal Septum. Obstet Gynecol. 1979;54:60–4.
3. Jain N, Gupta A, Kumar R, Minj A. Complete imperforate transverse vaginal septum with septate uterus: a rare anomaly. J Hum Reprod Sci. 2013;6(1):74–6.
4. Dilbaz B, Altinbas SK, Altinbas NK, Sengul O, Dilbaz S. Concomitant imperforate hymen and transverse vaginal septum complicated with pyocolpos and abdominovaginal fistula. Case Rep Obstet Gynecol. 2014;2014:1–4.
5. Deligeoroglou E, Deliveliotou A, Makrakis E, Creatsas G. Concurrent imperforate hymen, transverse vaginal septum, and unicornuate uterus: a case report. J Pediatr Surg. 2007;42(8):1446–8.
6. Ahmed S, Morris LL, Atkinson E. Distal mucocolpos and proximal hematocolpos secondary to concurrent imperforate hymen and transverse vaginal septum. J Pediatr Surg. 1999;34(10):1555–6.
7. Wierrani F, Bodner K, Spangler B, Grunberger W. "Z"-plasty of the transverse vaginal septum using Garcia's procedure and the Grunberger modification. Fertil Steril. 2003;79(3):608–12.
8. Laufer MR. Structural abnormalities of the female reproductive tract. In: Emans SJ, Laufer MR, editors. Emans, Laufer, Goldstein's pediatric and adolescent gynecology. 6th ed. Philadelphia: Lippincott Williams & Wilkins; 2012. p. 188–236.
9. Grimbizis GF, Gordts S, Di Seizio SA, Brucker S, De Angelis C, Gergolet M, et al. The ESHRE/ESGE consensus on the classification of female genital tract congenital anomalies. Hum Reprod. 2013;28(8):2032–44.
10. Grimbizis GF, Campo R. Congenital malformations of the female genital tract: the need for a new classification system. Fertil Steril. 2010;94(2):401–7.
11. Acien P, Acien MI. The history of female genital tract malformation classifications and proposal of an updated system. Hum Reprod Update. 2011;17(5):693–705.
12. Oppelt P, Renner SP, Brucker S, Strissel PL, Strick R, Oppelt PG, et al. The VCUAM (Vagina Cervix Uterus Adnex-associated Malformation) classification: a new classification for genital malformations. Fertil Steril. 2005;85(5):1493–7.
13. Williams CE, Nakhal RS, Hall-Craggs MA, Wood D, Cutner A, Pattison SH, Creighton SM. Transverse vaginal septae: management and long term outcomes. BJOG. 2014;121:1653–9.
14. Levy G, Warren M, Maidman J. Transverse vaginal septum: case report and review of the literature. Int Urogynecol J Pelvic Floor Dysfunct. 1997;8:173–6.
15. Banerjee R, Laufer MR. Reproductive disorders associated with pelvic pain. Semin Pediatr Surg. 1998;7(1):52–61.
16. Breech LL, Laufer MR. Mullerian anomalies. Obstet Gynecol Clin North Am. 2009;36:47–68.
17. Dietrich JE, Miller DM, Quint EH. Obstructive reproductive tract anomalies. J Pediatr Adolesc Gynecol. 2014;27:396–402.
18. Rock JA. Anomalous development of the vagina. Semin Rerpod Endocrinol. 1986;4:13–31.

19. Suidan FG, Azoury FS. The transverse vaginal septum: a clinicopathologic evaluation. Obstet Gynecol. 1979;54(3):278–83.
20. Simpson JL. Genetics of the female reproductive ducts. Am J Med Genet. 1999;89:224–39.
21. Slavotinek AM. Mckusick-Kaufman syndrome. Gene Review. http://www.ncbi.nlm.nih.gov/books/NBK1502/. Accessed 29 June 2010.
22. Ameh EA, Mshelbwala PM, Ameh N. Congenital vaginal obstruction in neonates and infants: recognition and management. J Pediatr Adolesc Gynecol. 2011;24:74–8.
23. Rock JA, Brrech LL. Surgery for anomalies of the mullerian ducts. In: Rock JA, Jones HW, editors. Telinde's operative gynecology. 10th ed. Philadelphia: Lippincott Williams & Wilkins; 2009. p. 539–84.
24. Attaran M, Falcone T, Gidwani G. Obstructive mullerian anomalies. In: Gidwani G, Falcone T, editors. Congenital malformations of the female genital tract. Philadelphia: Lippincott Williams & Wilkins; 1999. p. 145–68.
25. Rock JA, Azziz R. Genital anomalies in Childhood. Clin Obstet Gynecol. 1987;30(3):682–96.
26. Kaya C, Cengiz H, Ekin M, Yasar L. Transverse vaginal septum: a benign reason for elevated serum CA19-9 and CA 125 levels. Arch Gynecol Obstet. 2012;286:821–3.
27. Bermejo C, Martinez-Ten P, Recio M, Ruiz-Lopez L, Diaz D, Illescas T. Three-dimensional ultrasound and magnetic resonance imaging assessment of cervix and vagina in women with uterine malformations. Ultrasound Obstet Gynecol. 2014;43:336–45.
28. Krafft C, Hartin CW, Ozgediz DE. Magnetic resonance as an aid in the diagnosis of a transverse vaginal septum. J Pediatr Surg. 2012;47:422–5.
29. Church DG, Vancil JM, Vasanawala S. Magnetic resonance imaging for uterine and vaginal anomalies. Curr Opin Obstet Gynecol. 2009;21:379–89.
30. Olpin JD, Heilbrun M. Imaging of mullerian duct anomalies. Clin Obstet Gynecol. 2009;52(1):40–56.
31. Humphries PD, Simpson JC, Creighton SM, Hall-Craggs MA. MRI assessment of congenital vaginal anomalies. Clin Radiol. 2008;63:442–8.
32. Brown MA, Mattrey RF, Stamato S, Sirlin CB. MRI of the female pelvis using vaginal gel. AJR Am J Roentgenol. 2005;185:1221–7.
33. Lang IM, Babyn P, Oliver GD. MR imaging of paediatric uterovaginal anomalies. Pediatr Radiol. 1999;29:163–70.
34. Quint EH, McCarthy JD, Smith YR. Vaginal surgery for congenital anomalies. Clin Obstet Gynecol. 2010;53(1):115–24.
35. Van Bijsterveldt C, Willemsen W. Treatment of patients with congenital transversal vaginal septum or partial aplasia of the vagina. The vaginal pull-through versus the push-through technique. J Pediatr Adolesc Gynecol. 2009;22:157–61.
36. Bush NC, Prieto JC, Baker LA. Vaginoplasty in children using autologous buccal mucosa. J Urol. 2008;179(4):94.

37. Yesim Ozgenel G, Ozcan M. Neo vaginal construction with buccal mucosal grafts. Plast Reconstr Surg. 2003;111:2250–4.
38. Raya-Rivera AM, Esquiliano D, Fierro-Pastrana R, Lopez Bayghen E, Valencia P, Ordorica-Flores R, et al. Tissue-engineered autologous vaginal organs in patients: a pilot cohort study. Lancet. 2014;384: 329–36.
39. Lacy J, Correll GR, Walmer DK, Price TM. Simple vaginal mold for use in the postoperative care of patients with transverse vaginal septum. Fertil Steril. 2007;87(5):1225–6.
40. Hurst BS, Rock JA. Preoperative dilation to facilitate repair of the high transverse vaginal septum. Fertil Steril. 1992;57(6):1351–3.
41. Mizia K, Bennett MJ, Dudley J, Morrisey J. Mullerian dysgenesis: a review of recent outcomes at Royal Hospital for Women. Aust N Z J Obstet Gynaecol. 2006;46:29–31.
42. Dennie J, Pillay S, Watson D, Grover S. Laparoscopic drainage of hematocolpos: a new treatment option for the acute management of a transverse septum. Fertil Steril. 2010;94(5):1853–7.
43. Miller RJ, Breech LL. Surgical correction of vaginal anomalies. Clin Obstet Gynecol. 2008;52(2):223–36.
44. Beyth Y, Klein Z, Weinstein S, Tepper R. Thick transverse vaginal septum: expectant management followed by surgery. J Pediatr Adolesc Gynecol. 2004;17:373–81.
45. Burgis J. Obstructive mullerian anomalies: case report, diagnosis, and management. Am J Obstet Gynecol. 2001;185(2):338–44.
46. Rock JA, Zacur HA, Dlugi AM, Jones HW, TeLinde RW. Pregnancy success following surgical correction of imperforate hymen and complete transverse vaginal septum. Obstet Gynecol. 1982;59(4):448–51.
47. Malhotra V, Bhuria V, Nanda S, Chauhan MB, Dahiya P. Transverse vaginal septum in labor. J Gynecol Surg. 2013;29(4):207–9.
48. Blanton EN, Rouse DJ. Trial of labor in women with transverse vaginal septa. Obstet Gynecol. 2003; 101(5):1110–2.

Cervical Agenesis

5

Jovana Lekovich and Samantha M. Pfeifer

Definition

Cervical agenesis (Greek: *a*- without, γένεσησ= formation) is a rare congenital mullerian duct malformation characterized by complete failure of cervical development. It was first described by Ludwig in 1900. Manifestations of this anomaly include complete failure of development of cervical tissue (cervical agenesis) and variations in presence of some cervical tissue including normal cervical development with just distal occlusion, and fibrous band of tissue that can contain isolated areas of endocervical tissue [1] (Fig. 5.1). Cervical agenesis may be present with a normal or shortened vagina, but typically close to 50 % of the cases are associated with vaginal atresia/agenesis [2]. Although in the majority of cases the uterine configuration is normal, there may be associated uterine anomalies present. Uterus didelphys, bicornuate uterus, bicornuate uterus with obstructed horn, unicornuate uterus have all been reported in association with cervical agenesis [2–4]. The risk of renal anomalies seen with cervical agenesis is in the range of 10–25 %, but may vary with the type of uterine malformation seen [1, 2].

Incidence

The true incidence of cervical agenesis remains difficult to determine. By Buttram and Gibbons' classification scheme from 1979 [5] as well as its later revision by American Fertility Society in 1988 [6], isolated cervical agenesis represents a rare class IB mullerian anomaly. What makes the determination of incidence difficult using these two classifications is the fact that the Mayer-Rokitansky-Kuster-Hauser syndrome (also referred to as mullerian agenesis or mullerian aplasia), a relatively common uterine anomaly, is represented by various degrees of underdevelopment (and complete absence) of the uterus, cervix, and fallopian tubes and therefore can include cervical agenesis. Both of the classifications primarily focus on the uterus and vagina, disregarding the cervix and adnexa. The more recent classification by Oppelt et al. from 2005 [7]—so called VCUAM (Vagina Cervix Uterus Adnex-associated Malformation) classification—places cervical malformations in its own C class, with cervical agenesis representing the C2 subclass. As mentioned earlier, cervical agenesis may or may not be associated with vaginal atresia, a condition easier to diagnose and therefore with higher incidence. The incidence of vaginal atresia has been reported

J. Lekovich, M.D. (✉)
Ronald O. Perelman and Claudia Cohen Center for reproductive Medicine Weill Cornell Medical College, New York, NY, USA
e-mail: jol9105@med.cornell.edu

S.M. Pfeifer, M.D.
Weill Cornell Medical College, New York, NY 10021, USA
e-mail: spfeifer@med.cornell.edu

© Springer International Publishing Switzerland 2016
S.M. Pfeifer (ed.), *Congenital Müllerian Anomalies*, DOI 10.1007/978-3-319-27231-3_5

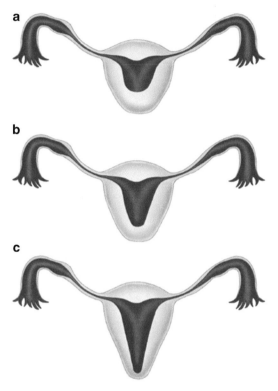

Fig. 5.1 Types of cervical agenesis/dysgenesis: (**a**) Complete failure of development of cervical tissue (cervical agenesis). (**b**) Presence of some cervical tissue (otherwise referred to as cervical dysgenesis). This distal cervical area is typically fibrous but may contain isolated islands of endocervical tissue. (**c**) Normal cervical development with distal occlusion

to be 1:4000 to 1:5000 [8, 9] with <10 % of these patients demonstrating cervical agenesis as well [10]. Consequently, in a series of 58 patients with congenital cervical agenesis, approximately 50 % had isolated cervical agenesis with normal vaginal development [11]. Overall, there are less than 100 cases of congenital cervical agenesis described in literature [1–3, 12–27].

Etiology

The etiology of cervical agenesis is not well understood. Our understanding of genetic components involved in normal development of the genital tract heavily relies on knockout animal models. The *Wnt* gene family has been implicated in sex determination and development of female reproductive tract. Wnt5a gene deficient female mice have been found

to have no cervical and vaginal development [28]. Homeobox family of genes, specifically homeobox A 9 (HOXA9), 10 (HOXA10), 11 (HOXA11), and 13 (HOXA13), are expressed along the paramesonephric ducts during early development and have been implicated in morphogenesis of the fallopian tubes, uterus, cervix, and vagina. Female mice with homozygous deletion of a 90-bp segment within the first exon of HOXA 13 demonstrate absence of cervical and vaginal cavity in addition to absence of digits [29].

The development of the female reproductive tract also depends on the effects of estrogen that is being produced by the fetal ovaries. Estrogen receptor (ER) α is more commonly expressed than ERβ [30]; however, ER α knockout mice have small but normally patterned reproductive tract. There are no reported cases of familiar cervical agenesis, and no particular gene mutations have been proposed.

Diagnosis

Unlike some other mullerian anomalies that can remain asymptomatic for a longer period of time, individuals with cervical agenesis most commonly present in early adolescence. It is either pelvic pain or primary amenorrhea that makes the parents or the patient seek evaluation. Pain is the most common presenting symptom and is due to menstrual blood accumulation in the uterus. Pain occurs shortly after menarche because the uterus is small and not distensible and therefore cannot accommodate a large amount of menstrual blood. Retrograde menstruation through the fallopian tubes occurs relatively quickly leading to pain, endometriosis, adhesions, and tubal occlusion. This is in contrast to the situation with an imperforate hymen, which presents much later after menarche as the vagina is distensible and able to accommodate a significant volume of menstrual blood before symptoms occur. Initially, the pain is typically sporadic or cyclic reflecting the regularity of the menstrual cycle in the post-menarcheal period. However, pain eventually becomes constant due to accumulation of blood within the uterus, fallopian tubes and development of endometriosis. Primary amenorrhea is not a common presenting symptom as the patients are typically very young at diagnosis (11–15 years old) and lack of menses might not be necessarily regarded as abnormal in this age group.

Physical exam may reveal abdominal tenderness, but unlike other obstructed anomalies, a mass may not be palpable because the uterus is not distensible and cannot accommodate a large amount of menstrual blood. If a mass is palpable, it is more likely to be a hematosalpinx or ovarian endometrioma occurring as a result of retrograde menstruation [27]. Associated upper tract findings include hematosalpinx, endometriosis, endometriomas, and pelvic adhesions (Table 5.1) [3, 31, 32]. Genital exam may reveal vaginal agenesis with a vaginal dimple or a blind ending vagina of variable lengths that does not connect to the uterus.

Transabdominal or transperineal ultrasound can generally be helpful in determining the level of the obstruction [33, 34]. Transrectal ultrasound might be able to detect cervical agenesis [35]; however, this exam is more invasive than a transabdominal approach. Unless a physician and a

radiologist have a high clinical suspicion for this condition, sonographic finding of hematometra can easily be mistaken for a pelvic mass, which can lead to misdiagnosis and surgery. MRI is the imaging modality of choice for diagnosis of this uterine anomaly as it can clearly demonstrate the absence or presence of the cervix, and can differentiate cervical agenesis from other conditions with similar presentation (such as high transverse vaginal septum) (Fig. 5.2) [11, 36, 37]. MRI can

Table 5.1 Associated upper tract findings in recent studies

	Deffarges	Fedele	Kriplani
	2001	2008	2012
# Patients	18	12	14
Hematosalpinx	11 %	83 %	14.2 %
Endometriosis: I, II	22 %	58 %	28.5 %
Endometriosis: III, IV	22 %	–	35.7 %
Adhesions	22 %	83 %	28.5 %
Vaginal agenesis	39 %	17 %	65 %
Cervical agenesis	Not reported	83 %	64.2 %
Cervical remnant/ dysgenesis		17 %	35.7 %

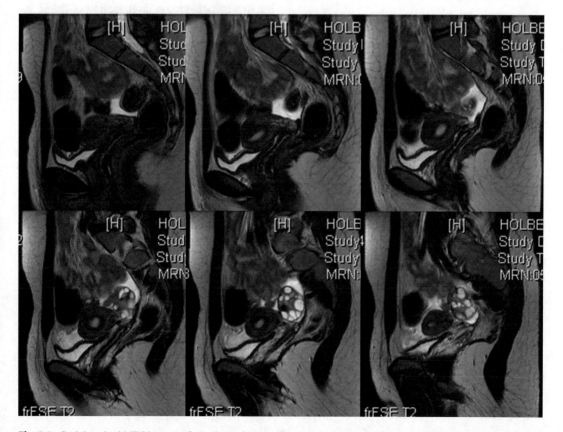

Fig. 5.2 Serial sagittal MRI images of a patient with complete cervical agenesis. Note no evidence of cervical tissue

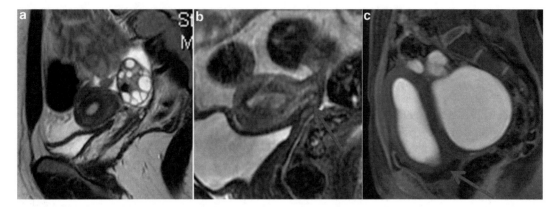

Fig. 5.3 MRI of 3 different patients with cervical agenesis. (**a**) Complete cervical agenesis. (**b**) Fibrous cervical tissue +/– endocervical glands (not typically visible on MRI). (**c**) Distal cervical occlusion. Note large hematosalpinx adjacent to the uterus, sequelae of delayed diagnosis

also demonstrate the degree of cervical agenesis and the size of the uterus which may be helpful in counseling the patient and her family about treatment options (Fig. 5.3). However, a clinician should be aware of this imaging modality's limitations in case of previous surgery [38].

Differential Diagnosis

The differential diagnosis for cyclic or episodic pain in a premenarcheal female in addition to cervical agenesis includes any other obstructed mullerian anomaly. High transverse vaginal septum and distal vaginal agenesis are the most similar in presentation to cervical agenesis because there is little room for menstrual blood to accumulate in a small vaginal cavity so the symptoms become more severe quickly and there is less likely to be a large mass palpable. Cervical agenesis must be distinguished from high transverse vaginal septum because treatment differs. The best way to differentiate these two conditions is with MRI to delineate the presence of a cervix and hematocolpos with the vaginal septum [36]. The cervix acts as a barrier to infection between the vagina and the upper genital tract and peritoneal cavity. This barrier is intact following resection of a transverse vaginal septum with anastomosis of upper and lower vaginal segments. However, in the absence of a cervix, anastomosis of vagina to uterus has resulted in ascending infection and

death [39]. Other obstructed mullerian anomalies such as low transverse vaginal septum and imperforate hymen have similar presentation and must be differentiated from cervical agenesis. However, in both of these conditions there is usually a large hematocolpos present, which may accumulate a significant amount of blood, resulting in a palpable mass on palpation of the abdomen and a longer time to diagnosis.

Treatment

When planning treatment for a patient with cervical agenesis the goals are relief of pain and considerations of future fertility. Traditionally, removal of the uterus has been the treatment of choice due to a significant risk of infection, morbidity, and death with attempts to salvage the uterus for future fertility [1, 40]. However, due to improved minimally invasive surgical procedures and developments in assisted reproductive technologies, alternative fertility sparing procedures have been considered. When deciding on the appropriate procedure for the individual patient, the following questions should be considered: (1) Is the uterus large enough to sustain a pregnancy; (2) Is there a cervical segment present (i.e., cervical dysgenesis vs. agenesis); (3) Is the vagina developed; and (4) Is the patient able to contribute to the decision-making process. If there are concerns about the best approach or the patient's ability to be involved in the decision-making process, then medical management may be utilized to defer definitive surgical treatment.

Removal of Uterus

Early studies evaluating surgical approaches to cervical agenesis compared hysterectomy to creation of a fistulous tract between the vagina and uterus. In one study of 18 patients, 13 were treated with creation of fistulous tract and five with primary hysterectomy [18]. Of those with fistulous tract approach, two underwent reoperation for occlusion, two underwent subsequent hysterectomy many years later, and one underwent hysterectomy with salpingo-oophorectomy with subsequent death due to sepsis. Another study of 30 patients, 11 underwent uterovaginal anastomosis with six of them subsequently undergoing reoperation for obstruction and infection and ultimately underwent hysterectomy [1]. Those who had cervical agenesis or cervical fragmentation were the cases who experienced the complications. Those who were successful with the uterovaginal anastomosis had a normally formed cervix with distal obstruction. The patients who underwent hysterectomy had no complications. Based on these studies, the recommendation was to remove the uterus in cases of cervical agenesis and most cases of cervical dysgenesis to avoid the risks and morbidity of reoperation for re-obstruction and infection.

Uterine Vaginal Anastomosis

Although the above reports suggested that uterovaginal anastomosis carried a high rate of reocclusion necessitating multiple surgical procedures and resulting in subsequent hysterectomy, some of those patients did have successful outcomes [1, 18, 40]. In addition there were case reports of pregnancies occurring after uterovaginal anastomosis, most in patients with partial cervical atresia or cervical dysgenesis [16, 23, 24, 41]. Some of these pregnancies were unassisted and some were the result of assisted reproductive technologies.

In one case series 40 % of those who attempted to become pregnant had a successful pregnancy [3]. Given these successes, fertility sparing surgery has been reconsidered.

More recently, several case series have described uterovaginal anastomosis for cervical agenesis with or without vaginal agenesis to preserve uterine function and fertility as an alternative to hysterectomy [3, 31, 32, 42]. In contrast to the earlier reports, these newer series have shown much better results with rare complications noted. In all the series, the majority of the patients had resumption of menses and vaginal adequacy with many sexually active without complication. Given the young age at the time of the initial surgery and short follow-up, not all patients were at an age to become sexually active. Two of the case series reported no complications in 18 and 12 patients, respectively [31, 42]. Restenosis was reported in the other two studies. In one series, restenosis was noted in 1/18 patients who required multiple canalization procedures, with subsequent infection and salpingo-oophorectomy [3]. In the other case series of 14 patients, there was 1 patient who had vaginal restenosis resulting in infection with tubo-ovarian abscesses requiring hysterectomy [32]. In these studies, pregnancies and live births have been reported. However, it is important to note that these excellent results published in these case series reflect treatment by skilled surgeons with experience in managing these anomalies. Uterovaginal anastomosis is a complex procedure with significant risks such as recurrent restenosis of the cervical canal, ascending infection, sepsis, and possible death [2, 39] and as such should be performed by an experienced surgeon.

The technique described in all these case series involved mobilizing the uterus from above either laparoscopically or at laparotomy, some including transection of the round ligaments to facilitate mobilization [2, 3, 26, 31]. An opening is then made from above into the uterus fundus through which a probe is placed through to the cervical area to facilitate mobilization and location of the uterus from below (Fig. 5.4). Dissection is then carried out from below to locate the uterus starting at the apex of the vagina,

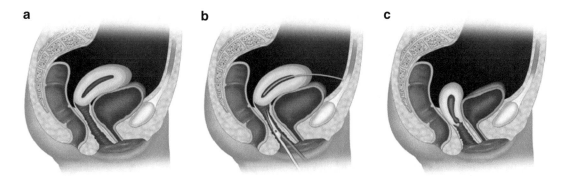

Fig. 5.4 Uterovaginal anastomosis: (**a**) Depicting uterus with cervical agenesis at apex of vaginal canal. (**b**) A probe is placed through the fundus of the uterus from above, applying pressure to facilitate mobilization and location of the uterus while dissection is carried out from below from the apex of the vagina through the tissue between the bladder and rectum. (**c**) An opening is made in the cervical area of the uterus from below: either by a single incision or a cone-biopsy like resection. The opened cervix is then anastomosed to the upper vaginal edges with interrupted delayed absorbable sutures

through the space between the rectum and bladder, while simultaneous downward pressure is exerted on the uterus from above with the uterine probe. Once the uterus is reached, an opening is made in the cervical area of the uterus from below: either by a single incision or a cone-biopsy like resection. The opened cervix is then anastomosed to the upper vaginal edges with interrupted delayed absorbable sutures. In most cases a silicone stent is placed extending from the vagina through the cervix into the uterus and sutured in place with delayed absorbable suture to maintain cervical patency.

and also for the adolescent who, at an older age, may better be able to participate in her own health care decisions. This is also a reasonable option to defer surgery in the case where a surgeon experienced in treating these complex anomalies is not immediately available. In addition, pregnancies have been reported in women with cervical atresia and cervical stenosis following surgical repair utilizing IVF with transmyometrial embryo transfer [43, 44]. In these cases, if the patient is asymptomatic, surgery may be deferred indefinitely as long as the risks of hormonal suppression are outweighed by the benefits.

Medical Suppression

An alternative to immediate surgical correction of this anomaly is to medically suppress menstruation to defer definitive surgical treatment till later. This may be accomplished with combined oral contraceptive pills given continuously, progestins including norethindrone acetate continuously, depo-medroxy progesterone, or GnRH agonist therapy with add-back. In cases where the individual is in extreme pain, laparoscopic drainage of the distended uterus can be performed first [2]. This option allows time to weigh the surgical options of hysterectomy versus fertility sparing uterovaginal anastomosis for the parents

Associated Vaginal Agenesis

Cervical agenesis with associated vaginal atresia or agenesis is a more complex condition as consideration must be made for lengthening or creating a neovagina. This can be accomplished at the same time as the surgery to address cervical agenesis or at a separate procedure. Options for simultaneous correction include utilizing a modified McIndoe approach where graft tissue is used to line the neovagina dissected space connecting the native vaginal tissue and the newly created cervical opening. Options for graft tissue include full split thickness skin graft, buccal mucosa, amnion, autologous in vitro-cultured vaginal tissue, and Interceed [45, 46]. Following placement of graft, a vaginal mold must be worn postoperatively until sexually active to prevent graft contracture. Rates of successful patency following uterovaginal canalization with vaginoplasty are lower than uterovaginal anastomosis alone: 43 % vs. 68 %, respectively [2]. Intestinal vaginoplasty using sigmoid colon in a patient with vaginal and cervical agenesis has been described [47]. Alternatively, vaginal dilation may be used to lengthen the vagina so that native vaginal tissue may be used. This process may take 6–9 months to achieve adequate vaginal length, so vaginal cervical anastomosis must be deferred, utilizing hormonal suppression of menses for pain control. If hysterectomy is the primary surgical procedure performed, then creation of neovagina or vaginal lengthening may be deferred until the patient is ready to address this. In this scenario, the patient would be treated as any other individual with vaginal agenesis with vaginal dilation considered the first choice of therapy.

Management Considerations

The decision regarding which procedure to perform is complex. Traditionally, hysterectomy was considered the best option for these individuals as vaginal utero anastomosis carries risks of reocclusion, infection, and multiple surgical procedures. However, loss of reproductive function is difficult for many individuals and therefore there is a role for procedures that spare reproductive function. There are many factors that should be considered in making this decision. The size of the uterus is important. If the uterus is very small, then it is less likely that it will be able to carry a pregnancy successfully and hysterectomy may be the better option. If the uterus is large, then pregnancy may be feasible and consideration should be made to preserve the uterus. However, it is important to note that with obstruction, the uterus may appear larger than it actually is due to distention of the uterine cavity and associated muscle hypertrophy. Presence of cervical tissue is probably also important. In the older literature, successful vaginal utero anastomoses

with pregnancies were reported primarily in those with cervical dysgenesis rather than agenesis [1]. However, in the recent studies, presence or absence of cervical tissue is not always noted, and it is not a factor in determining whether or not to proceed with uterovaginal anastomosis or pregnancy [3, 31, 32]. If cervical remnant tissue is present, that may be a more favorable condition for fertility preserving procedure. The absence of a vagina is another factor to consider in deciding which procedure to perform. Combining neovagina surgery with vaginal utero anastomosis is a more complicated procedure and is associated with additional risks for postoperative complications, such as vaginal stenosis, when compared to the single procedure and has been reported to have a poorer cervical patency rate [2]. For some individuals these risks may not outweigh the benefits. The patient's ability to contribute to the decision-making process is also important. Many young adolescents are not able to weigh the complexities, risks, and benefits of the surgical options and may not fully appreciate the concept of loss or preservation of reproductive function. For many of them immediate relief of pain is their major concern. Delaying the decision for definitive surgery in those cases where the uterus may be capable of carrying a pregnancy affords the individual the option to be part of the decision-making process at a more appropriate age. There may be some cases where the pain is so severe that suppression of menses is difficult or suppression may not result in adequate pain relief. In those cases surgery may not be deferred. In order to decide which procedure is appropriate for the individual, a thorough discussion with the patient and family is necessary. Issues to discuss include the surgical options, the risks of surgery, the postoperative risks of uterovaginal anastomosis such as reocclusion, infection, and subsequent surgical procedures, the likelihood of a successful pregnancy based on the appearance of the uterus, the desire to preserve reproductive function, and the possibility of deferring surgery to allow better participation of the individual in the decision process. Although hysterectomy is a safer option, it may not be the best option when the factors above are considered.

Impact on Fertility/Reproduction

Patients with congenital atresia or agenesis of the cervix have a risk of developing endometriosis, pelvic adhesions, and hematosalpinges as a result of the obstruction and retrograde menstruation and delay in diagnosis. These conditions are significant risk factors for infertility. It has been observed that individuals with a high transverse vaginal septum have a worse prognosis for fertility than individuals with imperforate hymen and this is directly attributed to the sequelae of retrograde menstruation [48]. In addition, other conditions that may affect fertility in these individuals include cervical factors as cervical mucus production may not be adequate following the anastomosis. In spite of these issues unassisted pregnancies have occurred following successful uterovaginal anastomosis [2, 3, 42]. Pregnancies have also occurred following the use of assisted reproductive techniques such as in vitro fertilization and zygote intra-fallopian tube transfer [3]. In patients who have restenosis of the cervix, successful pregnancies have occurred utilizing IVF with ultrasound guided transmyometrial transfer of embryos following hormonal suppression of menses [43, 44, 49, 50].

References

1. Rock JA, Roberts CP, Jones HW. Congenital anomalies of the uterine cervix: lessons from 30 cases managed clinically a common protocol. Fertil Steril. 2010;94:1858–63.
2. Fujimoto VY, Miller JH, Klein NA, Soules MR. Congenital cervical atresia: report of seven cases and review of the literature. Am J Obstet Gynecol. 1997;177:1419–25.
3. Deffarges JV, Haddad I, Musset R, Paniel BJ. Uterovaginal anastomosis in women with uterine cervix atresia: long-term follow-up and reproductive performance. A study of 18 cases. Hum Reprod. 2001;16:1772–5.
4. Bakri Y, Al-Sugair A, Hugosson C. Bicornuate nonfused rudimentary uterine horns with functioning endometria and complete cervical-vaginal agenesis: magnetic resonance diagnosis. Fertil Steril. 1992;58:620–1.
5. Buttram Jr VC, Gibbons WE. Müllerian anomalies: a proposed classification (An analysis of 144 cases). Fertil Steril. 1979;32:40–6.

6. The American Fertility Society. The American Fertility Society classifications of adnexal adhesions, distal tubal occlusion, tubal occlusion secondary to tubal ligation, tubal pregnancies, Mullerian anomalies and intrauterine adhesions. Fertil Steril. 1988;49: 944–55.
7. Oppelt P, Renner SP, Brucker S, Strissel PL, Strick R, Oppelt PG, Doerr HG, Schott GE, Hucke J, Wallwiener D, Beckmann MW. The VCUAM (Vagina Cervix Uterus Adnex-associated Malformation) classification: a new classification for genital malformations. Fertil Steril. 2005;84:1493–7.
8. Engstad JE. Artificial vagina. Lancet. 1917;37: 329–31.
9. Brayan AL, Nigro JA, Counseller VS. One hundred cases of congenital absence of the vagina. Surg Gynecol Obstet. 1942;129:361–7.
10. Griffin JE, Edwards C, Madden JD, Harrod M, Wilson JD. Congenital absence of the vagina: the Mayer-Rokitansky-Kuster-Hauser Syndrome. Ann Intern Med. 1979;85:224–36.
11. Markham SM, Parmley TH, Murphy AA, Huggins GR, Rock JA. Cervical agenesis combined with vaginal agenesis diagnosed by magnetic resonance imaging. Fertil Steril. 1987;48:143–5.
12. Sherwood M, Speed T. Congenital atresia of the cervix. Tex Med. 1941;37:215–9.
13. Rotter C. Surgical correction of the congenital atresia of the cervix. Am J Obstet Gynecol. 1958;76:643–6.
14. Zarou G, Acken H, Brevetti R. Surgical management of congenital atresia of the cervix. Am J Obstet Gynecol. 1961;82:923–8.
15. Geary W, Weed J. Congenital atresia of the uterine cervix. Obstet Gynecol. 1973;42:213–7.
16. Zarou G, Esposito J, Zarou D. Pregnancy following the surgical correction of the congenital atresia of the cervix. Int J Gynecol Obstet. 1973;11:143–6.
17. Maciulla G, Heine M, Christian C. Functional endometrial tissue with vaginal agenesis. J Reprod Med. 1978;21:373–6.
18. Dillon W, Mudaliar N, Wingate M. Congenital atresia of the cervix. Obstet Gynecol. 1979;54:126–9.
19. Monks P. Uterus didelphys associated with unilateral cervical atresia and renal agenesis. Aust N Z J Obstet Gynaecol. 1979;19:245–6.
20. Niver D, Barrett G, Jewelewicz R. Congenital atresia of the uterine cervix and vagina: three cases. Fertil Steril. 1980;33:25–9.
21. Valdes C, Malini S, Malinak L. Sonography in the surgical management of vaginal and cervical atresia. Fertil Steril. 1983;40:263–5.
22. Jacob J, Griffin W. Surgical reconstruction of the congenitally atretic cervix: two cases. Obstet Gynecol Surv. 1989;44:556–68.
23. Fraser I. Successful pregnancy in a patient with congenital partial cervical atresia. Obstet Gynecol. 1989;74:443–5.
24. Thijssen R, Hollander J, Willemsen W, van der Heyden P, van Dongen P, Rolland R. Successful

pregnancy after ZIFT in a patient with congenital cervical atresia. Obstet Gynecol. 1990;76:902–4.

25. Suganuma N, Furuhashi M, Moriwaki T, Tsukahara S, Ando T, Ishihara Y. Management of missed abortion in a patient with congenital cervical atresia. Fertil Steril. 2002;77:1071–3.

26. Creighton SM, Davies MC, Cutner A. Laparoscopic management of cervical agenesis. Fertil Steril. 2005;85:1510–3.

27. Nunley WC, Kitchin JD. Congenital atresia of the uterine cervix with pelvic endometriosis. Arch Surg. 1980;115:757–8.

28. Mericskay M, Kitajewski J, Sassoon D. Wnt5a is required for proper epithelial-mesenchymal interactions in the uterus. Development. 2004;131: 2016–72.

29. Warot X, Fromental-Ramain C, Fraulob V, Chambon P, Dollé P. Gene dosage-dependent effects of the Hoxa-13 and Hoxd-13 mutations on morphogenesis of the terminal parts of the digestive and urogenital tracts. Development. 1997;124:4781–91.

30. Grecco TL, Furlow JD, Duello TM. Immunodetection of estrogen receptors in fetal and neonatal female mouse reproductive tracts. Endocrinology. 1991;129:1326–32.

31. Fedele L, Bianchi S, Frontino G, Berlanda N, Montefusco S, Borruto F. Laparoscopically assisted uterovestibular anastomosis in patients with uterine cervix atresia and vaginal aplasia. Fertil Steril. 2008;89:212–6.

32. Kriplani A, Kachhawa G, Awasthi D, Kulsherestha V. Laparoscopic-assisted uterovaginal anastomosis in congenital atresia of uterine cervix: a follow up study. J Minim Invasive Gynecol. 2012;19:477–84.

33. Graham D, Nelson MW. Combined perineal-abdominal sonography in the evaluation of vaginal atresia. J Clin Ultrasound. 1986;14:735–8.

34. Scanlan KS, Pozniak MA, Fagerhom M, Shapiro S. Value of transperineal sonography in the assessment of vaginal atresia. Am J Roentgenol. 1990;154:545–8.

35. Fedele L, Portuese A, Bianchi S. Transrectal ultrasonography in the assessment of congenital vaginal canalization defects. Hum Reprod. 1999;14:359–62.

36. Reinhold C, Hricak H, Forstner R, Ascher SM, Bret PM, Meter WR, Semelka R. Primary amenorrhea: evaluation with MRI imaging. Radiology. 1997;203:383–90.

37. Letterie GS. Combined congenital absence of the vaginal and cervix. Diagnosis with magnetic resonance imaging and surgical management. Gynecol Obstet Invest. 1998;46:65–7.

38. Lang IM, Babyn P, Oliver GD. MR imaging of pediatric utero-vaginal anomalies. Pediatr Radiol. 1999; 29:163–70.

39. Casey CA, Laufer MR. Cervical agenesis: septic death after surgery. Obstet Gynecol. 1997;90:706–7.

40. Rock JA, Schlaff WD, Zacur HA, Jones HW. The clinical management of congenital absence of the uterine cervix. Int J Gynaecol Obstet. 1984;22:231–5.

41. Hampton HL, Meeks GR, Bates GW, Wiser WL. Pregnancy after successful vaginoplasty and cervical stenting for partial atresia of the cervix. Obstet Gynecol. 1990;76:900–1.

42. Chakravarty B, Konar H, Chowdhury NN. Pregnancies after reconstructive surgery for congenital cervicovaginal atresia. Am J Obstet Gynecol. 2000;183:421–3.

43. Anttila L, Penttila TA, Suikkari AM. Successful pregnancy after in-vitro fertilization and transmyometrial embryo transfer in a patient with congenital atresia of cervix. Hum Reprod. 1999;14:1647–9.

44. Lai T, Wu M, Hung K, Cheng Y, Chang F. Successful pregnancy by transmyometrial and transtubal embryo transfer after IVF in a patient with congenital cervical atresia who underwent uterovaginal canalization during Caesarean section. Hum Reprod. 2001;16:268–71.

45. Callans N, De Cuypere G, De Sutter P, Monstrey S, Weyers S, Hoebeke P, Cools M. An update on surgical and non-surgical treatment for vaginal hypoplasia. Hum Reprod Update. 2014;20:775–801.

46. Grimsby GM, Baker LA. The use of autologous buccal mucosa grafts in vaginal reconstruction. Curr Urol Rep. 2014;15:428.

47. Lima M, Ruggeri G, Randi B, Domini M, Gargano T, La Pergola E, Gregori G. Vaginal replacement in the pediatric age group: a 34-year experience of intestinal vaginoplasty in children and young girls. J Pediatr Surg. 2010;45:2087–91.

48. Rock JA, Zacur HA, Dlugi AM, Jones HW, TeLinde RW. Pregnancy success following surgical correction of imperforate hymen and complete transverse vaginal septum. Obstet Gynecol. 1982;59:448–51.

49. Huberlant S, Tailland ML, Poirey S, Mousty R, Ripart-Neveu S, Mares P, de Tayrac R. Congenital cervical agenesis: pregnancy after transmyometrial embryo transfer. J Gynecol Obstet Biol Reprod. 2014;43:521–5.

50. Xu C, Xu J, Gao H, Huang H. Triplet pregnancy and successful twin delivery in a patient with congenital cervical atresia who underwent transmyometrial embryos transfer and multifetal pregnancy reduction. Fertil Steril. 2009;91:e1–3.

Müllerian Agenesis: Diagnosis, Treatment, and Future Fertility

6

Jamie Stanhiser and Marjan Attaran

Incidence

Mayer-Rokitansky-Kuster-Hauser (MRKH) syndrome is a congenital condition characterized by the absence or underdevelopment of the uterus and vagina secondary to mullerian duct aplasia. After gonadal dysgenesis, it is the most common cause of primary amenorrhea, and occurs in 1 in 4000–5000 female births [1]. It is also referred to as mullerian aplasia (MA), mullerian agenesis, utero-vaginal aplasia, *congenital absence of the uterus and vagina* (CAUV), and various arrangements of the names from the eponymous authors of the syndrome.

MRKH syndrome is the most severe manifestation in the spectrum of mullerian duct dysplasias. In this condition the vagina fails to develop and the uterine structures are variable in presentation. The uterine horns are typically separate, and their appearance ranges from cordlike structures extending along the pelvic sidewall to uterine horn like structures that may or may not contain functional endometrial tissue. The distal fallopian tubes are usually preserved and are in their normal anatomic position attached to the ovaries. The ovaries are typically positioned high in the pelvis or even above the pelvis and may be missed on pelvic ultrasound (Figs. 6.1, 6.2 and 6.3). Its clear identification and categorization is crucial to its clinical diagnosis and management. Despite the existence of several different classification systems the American Fertility Society (AFS) classification of mullerian duct anomalies is the most commonly used system historically. Mullerian aplasia is categorized as Class I in the AFS system, which designates hypoplasia or agenesis of mullerian structures [2]. Specifically MRKH would be designated as class IA classification. In 2012, the European Society of Human Reproduction and Embryology (ESHRE) and the European Society for Gynaecological Endoscopy (ESGE) introduced a classification system designated by the acronym CONUTA, for *congenital uterine anomalies* [3]. MRKH syndrome is categorized into CONUTA class U5 for dysplastic/aplastic uterus, and subcategorized into U5a or U5b based on the presence of a uterine rudimentary horn with or without a cavity, respectively. This syndrome is also categorized via the Online Mendelian Inheritance in Man (OMIM) as 277000.

Almost half the patients with MRKH will have additional congenital anomalies [4]. MRKH patients can be further divided into three groups based on the existence of these associated anomalies [5]. Isolated mullerian aplasia is referred to as Typical or Type I MRKH syndrome (Table 6.1). Atypical MRKH is when

The original version of this chapter was revised.
An erratum to this chapter can be found at
DOI 10.1007/978-3-319-27231-3_13

J. Stanhiser, M.D. • M. Attaran, M.D. (✉)
Cleveland Clinic, 9500 Euclid Avenue, A/81,
Cleveland, OH 44195, USA
e-mail: attaram@ccf.org

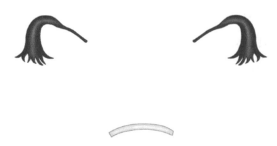

Fig. 6.1 MRKH with no discernable uterine structures. Distal fallopian tubes are usually present and attached to the ovaries

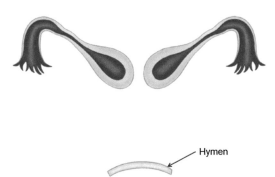

Hymen

Fig. 6.2 MRKH with absent vagina and two separate uterine horns each containing functional endometrial tissue. The uterine horns are usually on the lateral pelvic side walls

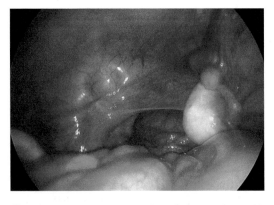

Fig. 6.3 Laparoscopic view of pelvis in a patient with MRKH. Note absence of uterus and position of ovaries high in pelvis. Fallopian tubes are present (image provided by Samantha M. Pfeifer M.D.)

the malformation is present not only in the uterus, but also in the ovary or the renal system. A particular constellation of anomalies is referred

Table 6.1 Classification of MRKH based on associated anomalies [5]

MRKH syndrome	Associated malformation
Typical	None
Atypical	Malformation of the ovary or renal system
MURCS	Malformation of the skeletal, cardiac, and renal system, muscular weakness

to as Type II MRKH syndrome or MURCS, for *m*ullerian duct aplasia, *r*enal aplasia, and *c*ervicothoracic *s*omite dysplasia, and occurs in more than one-third of cases [5]. Type II MRKH or MURCS is classified as OMIM 601076. The term *g*enital *r*enal *e*ar *s*yndrome (GRES) also can be used to describe a collection of these associated anomalies. In a study of 53 patients with MRKH, Oppelt and colleagues demonstrated that 47 % had typical form of MRKH, 21 % had the atypical form, and 32 % had the MURCS form of MRKH [5].

Anomalies of the renal system are the strongest associated malformations in patients with MRKH. Renal malformations include unilateral renal agenesis, renal ectopia including pelvic kidney, renal hypoplasia, or horseshoe kidney [6]. Cervicothoracic skeletal anomalies are the second most common malformation and include skeletal malformations such as scoliosis, fused or wedged vertebrae, and Klippel Feil anomaly (fusion of two or more cervical vertebrae, restriction of neck movement, a short neck, and low hair line). Less commonly, auditory defects are present and most commonly involve middle ear malformations leading to conductive deafness. Skeletal face and digital anomalies also can occur and include facial asymmetry, brachydactyly, syndactyly, polydactyly, and ectrodactyly. Cardiac anomalies have also been reported, and include aortopulmonary window, atrial septal defect, pulmonary valvular stenosis, and Tetralogy of Fallot. Additionally, Wottgen et al. in 2008 reported the incidence of associated anomalies in sibling and first-degree relatives of patients with MRKH is increased at 13 %. Particularly, skeletal and cardiac malformations in both sexes increased (3.27 and 2.3 times higher, respectively) from baseline risk in the normal population [7]. Interestingly, although renal malformations are the most common associated anomaly in patients with MRKH, their incidence is not increased from baseline in patient siblings.

Etiology

While the timing and pathway of embryologic development of the mullerian duct and structures associated with MURC anomalies are well understood, the exact etiology of MRKH syndrome remains mysterious despite extensive study.

The MURCS association of mullerian duct aplasia, renal dysplasia, and cervical somite anomalies, in addition to a broad spectrum of other associated anomalies, suggests a very distinct spatiotemporal moment in embryologic development when the embryonic cell precursors to all of these organ systems are related and vulnerable. This occurs at the end of the fourth week of embryonic development when blastemas of the lower cervical and upper thoracic somites and the pronephric ducts, which are the predecessor of the Wolffian duct and promote the mesonephron and Mullerian duct formation between 6 and 8 weeks, are interrelated. An affect at this stage of development would cause a cascade of anomalies and a developmental field defect. Several etiologic theories of embryologic environmental exposure to thalidomide similar teratogens or to altered levels of metabolites such as encountered in gestational diabetes and GALT deficiency galactosemia have been overturned despite initial observations of association [6, 7].

Neither does there appear to be a straightforward genetic explanation for this syndrome. Initially, isolated case reports of families in which two or three siblings all had mullerian agenesis gave credence to an autosomal dominant form of inheritance [7, 8]. However, the inability of women with this syndrome to reproduce made clear assessment of the inheritance pattern of MRKH difficult. The advent of in vitro fertilization and gestational surrogacy debunked the idea of strict autosomal dominant inheritance; to date none of the offspring of women with MRKH have had mullerian agenesis [9, 10] although one had an associated ear malformation causing deafness. Further discrediting the hypothesis of autosomal dominant inheritance, Wottgen et al. in 2008 assessed the siblings of 73 MRKH patients and no additional cases of MRKH occurred in any of the siblings, although siblings did have a 13 % incidence of associated anomalies. Additionally, case reports of discordant monozygotic twins in which one twin had MRKH and the other twin had either no abnormalities or an associated malformation such as a skeletal or cardiac anomaly but no mullerian abnormality suggest incomplete penetrance and high variable expressivity, and point to a more complicated, multifactorial etiology [7].

Several genes involved with embryological development including WT1, PAX2, HOXA7–HOXA13, PBX1, RAR-gamma, RXR-alpha, WNT4, and TCF2 have been studied for their possible role in MRKH syndrome, but evaluation has resulted in their vindication as causative factors. Interestingly when mutated, WNT4, which is involved with mullerian duct differentiation and nephrogenesis, results in a close but different and distinct syndrome of mullerian agenesis, hyperandrogenism and severe renal dysplasia collectively signified as WNT4 syndrome or WNT4 defects. Similarly, TCF2 mutation is very occasionally associated with mullerian agenesis only in the setting of maturity onset diabetes of the young (MODY) and renal dysplasia [6]. The gene encoding for the cystic fibrosis transmembrane regulator (CFTR) chloride channel has also been evaluated for the culpability of this syndrome, but no association has been found [11].

While women with MRKH typically have a normal karyotype of 46XX, extremely rare cases of X mosaicism and X deletion with gonadal dysgenesis and MRKH syndrome have been reported [12–14]. Additionally, in women with MRKH and a normal 46XX karyotype, small chromosomal deletions not visible on karyotype have been reported, without concordance between reports. One case report identified a chromosome 22 deletion in a patient with

MRKH syndrome [15]. Another case reported a chromosome 4 deletion in a patient with MRKH; however, the patient's mother had the same chromosomal deletion but normal mullerian anatomy with a cardiac defect [16]. This in combination with the previously presented literature argues strongly for a multifactorial, polygenic etiology of MRKH syndrome, which still remains unclear.

Differential Diagnosis

Patients with mullerian agenesis most commonly present as adolescents with normal growth and development. Secondary sexual characteristics develop in a timely manner; however, they have primary amenorrhea. On physical examination there is normal height, breast development, body hair, and external genitalia. However, the vagina is either entirely absent or present only as a short blind-ended pouch without a cervix at its apex. Other diagnoses that may share the same physical findings include vaginal atresia, transverse vaginal septum, and imperforate hymen. But most commonly this entity must be differentiated from Complete Androgen Insensitivity Syndrome (AIS).

History, physical examination, and pelvic imaging are the key to differentiating among these diagnoses. Patients are much more likely to present with cyclic or persistent pelvic and abdominal pain and/or a pelvic mass from hematocolpos in the case of lower vaginal atresia, transverse vaginal septum, or an imperforate hymen. These diagnoses are commonly not considered since the reproductive organs are not on the radar of clinicians caring for adolescents who have not yet begun to have menses. With some exceptions, individuals with MRKH and AIS will not complain of pelvic pain. Active endometrium in mullerian remnants has been reported in 2–7 % of patients with MRKH syndrome [17]. This subset of patients may therefore present with cyclic abdominal pain from hematometra, and cases have been reported of endometriosis from retrograde menstruation in obstructed uterine horns [17].

Physical examination can usually differentiate an obstructive anomaly from MRKH. Both will present with an apparent intact hymen on visual perineal exam. However, with imperforate hymen or transverse vaginal septum there may be a perineal bulge with valsalva or a hematometra which feels like a tense smooth mass palpable on rectal exam. With MRKH there is no mass from collected menstrual blood as the vagina and uterus are hypoplastic. Girls with MRKH will typically have age appropriate axillary and pubic hair, while girls with AIS typically have little or no pubic or axillary hair despite other signs of pubertal progression.

Pelvic ultrasound is usually the initial imaging technique utilized to investigate such patients. As noted above, the obstructive anomalies will show accumulation of blood in a cavity. This is not the case in patients with MRKH and AIS. In both of these diagnoses, a uterus is not seen although in some instances when the radiologist is not aware of the clinician's working diagnosis, the measurements of a very small rudimentary uterus may be noted in the report. This is very likely a measurement of the mullerian remnants in MRKH patients. The location of the ovaries is usually much higher in the pelvis of MRKH patients but in the same general area as in those with normal anatomy. The gonads in the AIS individual are detected in the abdomen at the point of entry into the inguinal canals, or in the inguinal canals and labia majora.

Hormone profiles and karyotype are paramount to distinguish MRKH syndrome from complete AIS. In girls with MRKH, serum total testosterone levels are within the normal range for females and the karyotype is 46XX. Individuals with AIS have a 46XY karyotype and typically have a serum total testosterone that is within the normal range for males. The testes in these individuals produce mullerian inhibiting substance (MIS) during fetal development resulting in regression of the mullerian structures. The testosterone and dihydrotestosterone produced, however, are ineffective in their function due to the androgen receptor defect. Thus these individuals will not develop male external genitalia and have diminished or absent axillary and pubic hair as the body will not respond to androgens produced from the adrenal gland during puberty. In addition, the testes in individuals with AIS are at risk for developing malignant tumors and current practice is to consider gonadectomy after puberty. Although there are structural similarities between these two conditions, it is important to differentiate MRKH from AIS as the management differs with regards to gonadectomy and counseling for issues of gender identity as well as fertility options.

Diagnosis

Given its high incidence, this diagnosis should be considered in any adolescent who presents with normal growth and development of secondary sexual characteristics but lack of menarche by age 16. On history the adolescent has usually progressed though the normal milestones of puberty with the exception of menses. Careful questioning may reveal the occurrence of cyclic pelvic pain reflecting ovulation (mittelschmerz). History will help to rule out other causes of amenorrhea such as energy deficit, prior exposure to gonadotoxic agents or other medications, dietary changes or any other systemic illnesses.

On examination, breasts may have developed to tanner 4–5 stage based on timing of presentation. Axillary and pubic hair will be normal. On examination the external genitalia will be normal in appearance and the area will be well estrogenized. As MRKH is the second most common cause of amenorrhea after gonadal dysgenesis, at a minimum, a q tip should be lightly applied to the vaginal opening to determine its length. The length of this vaginal pouch can be quite variable from a few mm to the full length of a normal vagina. If examination fails to show a vaginal opening or shows only a blind ending vaginal pouch, a pelvic ultrasound should be performed to determine if a uterus and ovaries are seen. Uterine agenesis or the presence of atrophic uterine horns with or without functional endometrial tissue can be confirmed with a magnetic resonance image (MRI) of the pelvis (Fig. 6.4). In addition, the MRI can locate the ovaries and evaluate the renal system. As 53 % of patients will have associated anomalies, it is important to always evaluate for linked congenital malformations. Additionally, given the increased incidence of associated malformations in siblings of patients with MRKH, patient family members should be evaluated for linked malformations [7].

Laparoscopy is not necessary for the diagnosis unless the patient has pain attributed to functioning endometrial tissue in the remnants. Laboratory evaluation reveals a normal female hormone profile, and normal 46XX karyotype.

Fig. 6.4 MRI of pelvis in a patient with MRKH showing absent uterine and vaginal structures (image provided by Samantha M. Pfeifer M.D.)

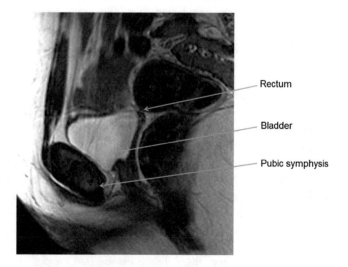

Rectum

Bladder

Pubic symphysis

Treatment

The goals of therapy are to reassure the patient regarding her well-being, her hormonal status, create a functioning vaginal canal for intercourse, and address issues pertaining to fertility.

Method of Delivering the Diagnosis to Patient

As would be expected this diagnosis is almost always unexpected. The adolescent who wants to be like her peers is automatically set apart from them in an unimaginable way. Thus the delivery of this information requires significant tact and thoughtfulness. The range of emotions that may be felt includes confusion, fear, depression, and ultimately isolation [18]. These patients must be seen routinely in the office to provide continued support and information to them. Psychological support must be offered, as failure to do so may lead to long-lasting psychological distress. Liao and colleagues had 56 MRKH patients' complete questionnaires on psychosexual wellness, emotional distress, and health related quality of life. Uniformly all the MRKH patients exhibited greater sexual anxiety and fear of sexual relations [19]. Education is an ongoing process with these patients and their parents. This may be obtained from repeated encounters with the physician but also by connecting them with specific educational web sites and support groups.

Creation of the Vagina

Throughout the years, numerous nonsurgical and surgical methods to create a vagina have been described (Table 6.2). There are few studies comparing the outcome of the various modalities of therapy with each other. In most instances the least invasive type of therapy is recommended. The patient's cultural and emotional background will also play a role in selecting the most suitable therapy. For instance there are patients that consider touching themselves a taboo and thus use of serial dilators would not be acceptable to

Table 6.2 Methods of creation of vaginal canal

Vaginal dilation	Intermittent pressure (Frank)
	Bicycle Seat (Ingram)
Dissection of perineal space	
• No graft	Insertion of balsa wood (Wharton)
• Split thickness skin graft	With use of mold (McIndoe)
• Autologous in vitro cultured vaginal tissue	Panici PB [37]
• Peritoneum	With use of mold (Davydov)
• Bowel	Use of sigmoid (Pratt)
• Muscle and skin flap	Modified Singapore (Woods)
Vulvovaginal pouch	Williams, Creatsas [40, 41]
Traction on the retrohymenal space	Vecchietti and Brucker [42]

them. Of course the training and experience of the operating physician will dictate the type of surgical therapy selected. Finally associated congenital anomalies and prior therapies will have an impact on the type of therapy that is chosen. Prior to creation of the vagina, it must be clear that the patient is emotionally and physically ready to care for the newly formed vagina. She must understand that dilators will be used after surgical therapy. The best functional outcome is obtained when the patient has to undergo only one surgery and is able to maintain the integrity of the newly created vagina.

All of the methods mentioned in Table 6.2 are still used today. However the majority are performed with various modifications from the original description. Some of them have been modified to be able to perform laparoscopically with newer instruments.

Vaginal Dilation

Vaginal dilation is considered the first line of therapy in the United States and United Kingdom. In 2013 American College of Obstetrics and Gynecology recommended use of vaginal dilation as the best option for creation of a vaginal canal in patients with mullerian agenesis [20]. There are two methods that are used for vaginal dilation. Most studies have been performed with

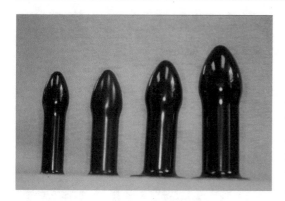

Fig. 6.5 Vaginal dilators in graduated lengths and widths used for vaginal lengthening. Dilators may come with conical or blunt tips and can be made of different materials (image provided by Samantha M. Pfeifer M.D.)

diagnosis and the general existing knowledge of infertility [23].

The complications noted with vaginal dilation may be inadvertent dilation of the urethra and vaginal prolapse. The former may be minimized by an inpatient therapy that is advocated in the United Kingdom, or by very frequent monitoring on an outpatient basis. Vaginal prolapse has been noted in both surgical and nonsurgically created vaginas. Prolapse has been documented to occur as early as during the process of dilation [24] or many years subsequent to this event [25]. The etiology is not clear, although some believe prolapse of the neovagina occurs because of lack of support at the apex of the new vagina.

intermittent application of a dilator to the perineum (Fig. 6.5). The patient applies the tip of the dilator to the opening within the hymen and applies a posteriorly directed pressure for 20–30 min at a time twice a day. Success rates have been quoted to range from 90 to 95 % [21, 22]. Some patients find it difficult to make the time to perform this task and maintain this awkward position. In such instances the Ingram method of dilation may be better suited to such individuals. They are instructed to apply the dilator to the perineum and then keep pressure applied by wearing a tight garment such as bicycle shorts. They can then sit on the dilator in a slightly tilted forward position on a bicycle seat or any hard chair. They then have their hands free to proceed with other tasks while dilation is taking place. Once one dilator fits easily into place then the next size dilator is used. Depending on the duration and frequency of dilation, a functioning vaginal length may be created in 4–11 months [22].

Most studies on vaginal dilation consider the process a success when the vaginal length is greater than 6 cm. Nadarajah and colleagues used the female sexual function index to measure the sexual functioning in 6 domains in 60 patients with mullerian agenesis who underwent vaginal dilation. While no difference was noted in arousal and desire, there was a difference in amount of lubrication and pain that was experienced in women with mullerian agenesis compared to controls. Factors that may contribute to this data are the patient's anxiety pertaining to her

Dissection of the Perineal Space

Creation of the perineal pouch was first described in 1835 [26]. Subsequent to this report several other techniques were explored, the primary theme being use of a lining on the newly created pouch and the ensuing prolonged use of a dilator. Ultimately the McIndoe technique gained popularity for many years [27]. Since that time many different types of tissues have been utilized to line the newly created cavity. These include skin, peritoneum, amnion, autologous in vitro cultured vaginal tissue, buccal mucosa, artificial grafts, and bowel. In the following section the technique for creation of this vaginal space will be described. In subsequent sections the issues pertaining to the specific lining agent will be discussed.

McIndoe Technique

Patient is placed in the dorsolithotomy position and a Foley catheter is placed in the bladder. A transverse incision is made on the perineum. Using fingers and dilators two canals are created and extended cephalad up to the peritoneum. If in the correct space, minimal amount of bleeding is encountered. Next the median raphe in between these canals is transected and any bleeding sites are controlled. At this time the cavity can now be lined by the designated tissue (Fig. 6.6). In our institution, the plastic surgery team obtains the skin graft. This may be obtained from the thighs or the buttocks. The skin graft is sutured around the mold using 4-0 absorbable suture, making

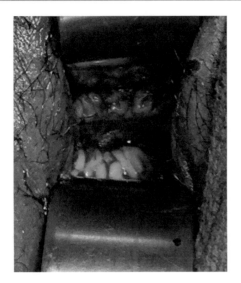

Fig. 6.6 Vaginal space after dissection between bladder and rectum and lined with buccal mucosa (image provided by Samantha M. Pfeifer M.D.)

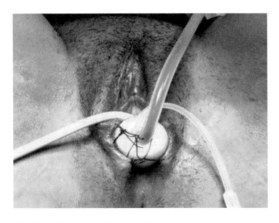

Fig. 6.7 Vaginal mold sutured in place after placement of graft tissue into neovagina dissected space (image provided by Samantha M. Pfeifer M.D.)

sure the dermal side will be in contact with the vaginal wall. The mold is then placed inside the newly created space and 4-0 absorbable suture is used to attach the skin graft to the vaginal opening/incision. The labia are sutured together over the mold with 2-0 silk loosely to keep the mold from falling out (Fig. 6.7).

During the next week the patient remains in bed to give time for the graft to adhere to the vaginal walls. The Foley catheter is in place, she is on a low residue diet, is maintained on antibiotics

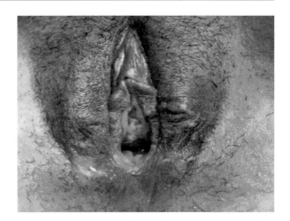

Fig. 6.8 One week after McIndoe procedure, patient is taken back to the operating room and the vaginal mold is removed, the neovagina irrigated and assessed for take of graft (image provided by Samantha M. Pfeifer M.D.)

and she is given an agent to slow bowel motility. After a week she returns to the operating room and has the mold carefully removed and the area lavaged (Fig. 6.8). The graft is assessed and any extra necrotic tissue is trimmed and removed. A new mold is now put in place. There are many different types of molds and none has been proven superior to others. We usually use a hard mold at the time of the first surgery and then a soft mold afterwards. The mold must be used continuously for the next 3 months. It may be removed with urination and defecation and then replaced. After this time, if she is not sexually active, it is recommended that she continue with use of the dilator at least at night time for the next 6 months.

The success rates for this surgery are 80 %. Although complications have decreased as more experience has been gained, they still can occur and include failure of graft take, infection and hemorrhage and fistula formation. However, the primary concern with this surgery is continued contracture of the vagina if a mold is not used or sexual activity is not consistent.

To combat this problem, some have advocated using full thickness skin grafts. Numerous techniques have been utilized through the years. Tissue expanders have been used in the labia to increase the length of this tissue and use it to line the vagina. Others have dissected the tissue on the vaginal dimple while still maintaining a connection posteriorly. The posterior vaginal wall is then lined by this tissue that is native to the area, has good blood supply, and has full thickness [28]. Others have advocated gracilis myocutaneous flaps and pudendal thigh flaps.

Agents Used to Line the Canal

Since the skin graft has the obvious disadvantage of leaving behind a scarred area on the body, other agents have been utilized throughout the years. In 1984 Dhall demonstrated that 10 weeks after placement of amnion into the neovaginal canal, the resulting epithelial tissue was indistinguishable from normal vaginal tissue histologically [29]. However it has the possibility of transmitting viral particles and thus it has not gained popularity. In more recent years agents such as buccal mucosa [30], oxidized cellulose [31], artificial dermis [32], and autologous in vitro cultured vaginal tissue [33] have been utilized to line the neovagina. In a recent study, Panici and colleagues reported on the outcome of use of autologous in vitro cultured tissue in 23 women with mullerian agenesis [34]. Patients first underwent a full thickness mucosal biopsy of the vaginal vestibule. This 1 cm^2 tissue is then dissociated and then cultured to ultimately obtain a fully differentiated mucosal tissue. This process may take up to 2–3 weeks. The gauze containing the cells is placed in the newly created vaginal canal and a dilator is put in place. After 5 days the dilator is removed and the vaginal canal is assessed. Vaginal tissue was noted to cover 70–100 % of the vaginal wall. In the initial 6 weeks after the operation the patient is advised to keep the dilator in place continuously until she is sexually active. Buccal mucosa has also been utilized in lining the surgically created vaginal space [35]. The advantages of buccal mucosa include lack of hair bearing epithelium, donor site scars that are hidden within the mouth, and minimal graft shrinkage. In addition buccal mucosa is very similar histologically to vaginal mucosa as both are nonkeratinized stratified squamous epithelium and therefore identical in color texture to native vaginal tissue. Buccal mucosa is typically harvested from both cheeks fenestrated, and sutured in place in a similar fash-

ion to a skin graft [35]. Alternatively, micromucosal grafting has been described where buccal mucosal cheek grafts are minced into tiny pieces and spread on gelatin sponge which are then used to create the neovaginal walls [36]. Reported success is similar to traditional McIndoe techniques [35, 36].

Davydov Technique

Another agent that has been used successfully to line the newly created perineal space is peritoneum. Its primary advantage over skin graft is that it avoids scarring on the body. This was first described by Davydov in 1969 [37]. In more recent years the laparoscopic modification has been used extensively. Although this technique may be used on any patient, it is more suitable for the patient that has had prior surgery on the perineum. Prior pelvic surgery might be construed a relative contraindication as there is a portion of this surgery that is performed intra-abdominally. During laparoscopy, the peritoneum in the pelvis is mobilized to such an extent that it can be pulled down into the newly created neovagina. The peritoneal margins are stitched to the mucosa of the perineum. Purse string stitches are applied to the peritoneum to form the most cephalad portion of the vagina and a dilator is kept in place postsurgically to prevent scarring. In a review of 30 patients undergoing this procedure, the average depth of the vagina was 7–8 cm and the mean hospital stay was 3.9±1.4 days [38]. Reported complications include intraoperative bladder and ureter injury, urinary retention, vesicovaginal fistulas, and hematoma of the anterior wall of the rectum.

Bowel Vaginoplasty

This technique is more commonly used in patients with complex cloacal abnormalities. However it may be utilized in MRKH patients that have failed other methods of vaginoplasty. Typically the sigmoid colon is mobilized on its vascular pedicle and is placed into the pelvis and connected to the introitus. Its major advantage is that it does not need continued dilation and it is well lubricated. However in some instances the mucous production is excessive leading to use of pads. In addition these individuals may develop intrinsic bowel disease or diversion colitis in the sigmoid neovagina. Its disadvantages are clear in that it is a significantly more invasive surgery than the other surgeries described in this chapter. In a recent systematic review of sexual function, bowel vaginoplasty was associated with longest vaginal length (12.87 cm), but more numerous complaints of dyspareunia and stenosis than other vaginoplasty methods [39].

Vulvovaginal Pouch

Williams vulvovaginoplasty was first described in 1964 [40]. The Creatsas modification has been described more recently in over 100 patients in which the origin of the incision on the labia majora is lower than originally described in William's vulvovaginoplasty [41]. After placement of a Foley in the bladder, an incision is made on the labia majora about 4 cm lateral to the urethra and carried downward and on to the perineum and then upward to the other labia majora in a U-shaped incision. The perineal tissue is mobilized and the inner skin margins of the incision are approximated with 2-0 incisions. Next the subcuticular tissue and muscles are approximated and finally the outer skin margins are approximated with the same suture. This procedure has the advantage of taking less time than some of the other surgical procedures, although the authors report a mean hospitalization time of 6 days. Its major advantage is that postoperative use of dilators is not necessary. Complications may include hematoma formation, wound dehiscence, and infection. After the area is fully healed the patient may attempt intercourse in this newly created pouch. Some have expressed concern over the axis of the newly created vagina.

Traction on the Retrohymeneal Space

The Vecchietti technique is considered to be a surgical version of "Frank's method." In 2008 Brucker and colleagues published their laparoscopic modification of the Vecchietti technique [42]. Instead of the initial creation of a space between the rectum and the bladder, an applicator is pushed through the perineum through the vesicorectal septum into the peritoneal cavity during laparoscopic observation. Attached to this

applicator are threads that are connected to a dilator. Once the treads are in the abdominal cavity, another curved applicator that has been placed through the abdominal wall is guided down retroperitoneally on the right and left pelvic side walls, until it reaches these threads. The threads are then loaded via laparoscopy into these applicators and gently withdrawn through the abdominal wall. The threads are then connected to an FDA approved traction device, kept on the abdominal wall, that can be tightened daily thereby pulling on the dilator on the perineum (Fig. 6.9). Within days a vaginal cavity is created as this device is tightened daily. However analgesia is necessary during this time (many use a continuous epidural delivery of analgesia) and patients must continue to use the dilator after the full vaginal length is developed. Brucker and colleagues have reported on the outcome of such a surgery on 101 patients. Average vaginal length was reported to be 9 cm and duration of hospital stay was 8.5 days. The

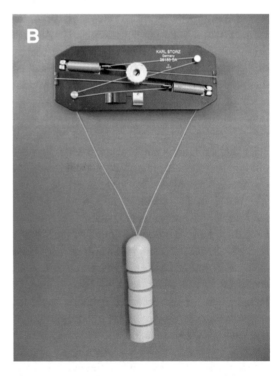

Fig. 6.9 Vecchietti traction device and vaginal "dummy." The large device is placed on the abdomen and the dummy is placed in the vagina with the traction wires passed subperitoneally through to the abdominal wall to the traction device [43]

mean duration of traction was 4.5 days. After creation of the vagina, the use of a dilator is recommended for a minimum of 6 months although sexual activity can start within 3 weeks. A more recent study from the same group describes the long-term outcome of 240 patients with MRKH who underwent this procedure [44]. Long-term follow-up (defined as ≥11 months) was available in 153 patients. Mean functional vaginal length was 9.5 cm, with a range of 6–13 cm, and epithelialization was 93 %. Compared to an age matched normal population, the female sexual function index scores (FSFI) of these patients were very similar.

Contraindications to this surgery would be prior vaginal surgery or exposure to radiation. Complications reported with this surgery are postoperative fever, urinary tract infections, hematoma of the bladder, and necrosis of the urethra [42].

Impact on Fertility and Reproduction

With the diagnosis of MRKH, a young woman learns not only that she lacks a functional vagina and uterus, but also that she cannot have intercourse without medical intervention, and she cannot carry a pregnancy herself. All three of these things she had previously considered a part of her identity as a female, and she learns of their absence in the setting of her adolescent psychological development. Incontestably, in addition to managing her anomaly medically, the enormous psychological aspects of this condition must be addressed and mitigated.

Following the diagnosis of MRKH syndrome, women experience shock, reactive depression, and enduring psychological distress that studies liken to the experience of trauma [18]. Acceptance and peace with their condition and their self-identity have been found to improve with time, and are increased in patients who receive psychological therapy in addition to medical therapy. Notable improvement has been reported in patients who receive counseling, cognitive behavioral therapy, and supportive group therapy [18].

Despite counseling, the lingering effects of this diagnosis are noted in many aspects of a patient's life. Although with time she realizes that the vagina is functioning and that her anatomy will be perceived as normal externally, the knowledge that her vagina is different can impact her perception of sex. Morcel and colleagues compared the functional outcome of intercourse in women with surgical versus nonsurgical methods of vaginal creation. The functional sexual results were similar in both groups. Scores were lower in the area of comfort and lubrication, leading one to extrapolate that the general anxiety an MRKH patient may experience can impact these parameters.

Although not persistently discussed in the beginning, the lack of ability to carry a child is haunting for many an adolescent and young woman. It is imperative that the health care provider explore this topic and offer options such as adoption and surrogacy. The concept of surrogacy may help temper the shock of the initial diagnosis as it provides the individual with the option to have one's own genetic child. In western culture this is certainly a viable option even though the various states and countries have differing laws. It is an expensive and exhaustive venture to find and recruit a surrogate and navigate the legal system. Women however may be reassured that the offspring of women with MRKH have not had MRKH themselves [9, 10]. Petrozza et al. in 1997 reported that out of 34 live-born children from gestational surrogacy there were no cases of MRKH in the female infants and no congenital anomalies except a middle ear defect causing conductive deafness in one male child. As noted earlier the location of the ovaries in some patients is higher and more lateral. Thus retrieval of oocytes may be more difficult in MRKH patients and less number of oocytes may be retrieved. Another potential problem is that women with atypical MRKH need more gonadotropins for a longer duration compared to other women. There is a report that women with the atypical form of MRKH did not stimulate as robustly as women with typical MRKH although the pregnancy rates in the two groups were similar [45].

While surrogacy is legal in the United States, in many countries surrogacy is illegal and some religions forbid its use. This limits the options for women with MRKH from some parts of the world. The concept of uterine transplantation has been under investigation for the past 10 years. It is really the only hope for reproduction for some women with mullerian agenesis. In 2013, a 35-year-old woman with MRKH syndrome underwent uterine transplantation from a living postmenopausal donor. Previous to the transplant, the patient underwent IVF and embryos were frozen for expected transfer, which was done 1 year after uterine transplantation. She became pregnant following her first single embryo transfer, and had a normal uncomplicated pregnancy until 31 weeks and 5 days estimated gestational age, at which time she developed preeclampsia and was delivered by cesarean section. The infant was born with APGAR scores of 9 and 9, and was discharged from the neonatal unit 16 days later in robust health [46].

There are many concerns that need to be further explored with uterine transplantation. Use of a uterus from a deceased individual would be associated with far less risk than harvesting a uterus from a live donor. This surgery involves extensive vasculature dissection in order to preserve vessels for re-anastomosis in the donor thereby placing the live donor at considerable risk. Another key issue is the length of time the MRKH patient should keep the uterus and be maintained on immunosuppressive therapy. In the above cited article, the patient was counseled regarding removal of the uterus after two deliveries. But who makes the definitive decision for a hysterectomy and when, remains a difficult question to answer. For now, uterine transplantation remains a viable hope for reproduction for some women with mullerian agenesis.

References

1. Patnaik SS, Brazile B, Dandolu V, Ryan PL, Liao J. Mayer-Rokitansky-Kuster-Hauser (MRKH) syndrome: A historical perspective. Gene. 2015; 555(1):33–40.
2. The American Fertility Society classifications of adnexal adhesions, distal tubal occlusion, tubal occlusion secondary to tubal ligation, tubal pregnancies, mullerian anomalies and intrauterine adhesions. Fertil Steril 1988;49(6):944–955.
3. Grimbizis GF, Gordts S, Di Spiezio SA, Brucker S, De Angelis C, Gergolet M, et al. The ESHRE/ESGE consensus on the classification of female genital tract congenital anomalies. Hum Reprod. 2013; 28(8):2032–44.
4. Oppelt PG, Lermann J, Strick R, Dittrich R, Strissel P, Rettig I, et al. Malformations in a cohort of 284 women with Mayer-Rokitansky-Kuster-Hauser syndrome (MRKH). Reprod Biol Endocrinol. 2012;10:57.
5. Oppelt P, Renner SP, Kellermann A, Brucker S, Hauser GA, Ludwig KS, et al. Clinical aspects of Mayer-Rokitansky-Kuester-Hauser syndrome: recommendations for clinical diagnosis and staging. Hum Reprod. 2006;21(3):792–7.
6. Morcel K, Camborieux L. Programme de Recherches sur les Aplasies Mulleriennes, Guerrier D. Mayer-Rokitansky-Kuster-Hauser (MRKH) syndrome. Orphanet J Rare Dis. 2007;2:13.
7. Wottgen M, Brucker S, Renner SP, Strissel PL, Strick R, Kellermann A, et al. Higher incidence of linked malformations in siblings of Mayer-Rokitansky-Kuster-Hauser-syndrome patients. Hum Reprod. 2008;23(5):1226–31.
8. Griffin JE, Edwards C, Madden JD, Harrod MJ, Wilson JD. Congenital absence of the vagina. The Mayer-Rokitansky-Kuster-Hauser syndrome. Ann Intern Med. 1976;85(2):224–36.
9. Petrozza JC, Gray MR, Davis AJ, Reindollar RH. Congenital absence of the uterus and vagina is not commonly transmitted as a dominant genetic trait: outcomes of surrogate pregnancies. Fertil Steril. 1997;67(2):387–9.
10. Beski S, Gorgy A, Venkat G, Craft IL, Edmonds K. Gestational surrogacy: a feasible option for patients with Rokitansky syndrome. Hum Reprod. 2000; 15(11):2326–8.
11. Timmreck LS, Gray MR, Handelin B, Allito B, Rohlfs E, Davis AJ, et al. Analysis of cystic fibrosis transmembrane conductance regulator gene mutations in patients with congenital absence of the uterus and vagina. Am J Med Genet A. 2003;120A(1):72–6.
12. Gardo S, Papp Z, Gaal J. XO-XX Mosaicism in the Rokitansky-Kuster-Hauser syndrome. Lancet. 1971;2(7738):1380–1.
13. Aydos S, Tukun A, Bokesoy I. Gonadal dysgenesis and the Mayer-Rokitansky-Kuster-Hauser syndrome in a girl with 46, X, del(X)(pter → q22:). Arch Gynecol Obstet. 2003;267(3):173–4.
14. Guven A, Kara N, Saglam Y, Gunes S, Okten G. The Mayer-Rokitansky-Kuster-Hauser and gonadal dysgenesis anomaly in a girl with 45, X/46, X, del(X)(p11.21). Am J Med Genet A. 2008;146A(1):128–31.
15. Cheroki C, Krepischi-Santos AC, Rosenberg C, Jehee FS, Mingroni-Netto RC, Pavanello Filho I, et al.

Report of a del22q11 in a patient with Mayer-Rokitansky-Kuster-Hauser (MRKH) anomaly and exclusion of WNT-4, RAR-gamma, and RXR-alpha as major genes determining MRKH anomaly in a study of 25 affected women. Am J Med Genet A. 2006;140(12):1339–42.

16. Bendavid C, Pasquier L, Watrin T, Morcel K, Lucas J, Gicquel I, et al. Phenotypic variability of a 4q34 → qter inherited deletion: MRKH syndrome in the daughter, cardiac defect and Fallopian tube cancer in the mother. Eur J Med Genet. 2007;50(1):66–72.

17. Cho MK, Kim CH, Oh ST. Endometriosis in a patient with Rokitansky-Kuster-Hauser syndrome. J Obstet Gynaecol Res. 2009;35(5):994–6.

18. Bean EJ, Mazur T, Robinson AD. Mayer-Rokitansky-Kuster-Hauser syndrome: sexuality, psychological effects, and quality of life. J Pediatr Adolesc Gynecol. 2009;22(6):339–46.

19. Liao LM, Conway GS, Ismail-Pratt I, Bikoo M, Creighton SM. Emotional and sexual wellness and quality of life in women with Rokitansky syndrome. Am J Obstet Gynecol. 2011;205(2):117.e1–6.

20. Committee on Adolescent Health Care. Committee opinion: no. 562: mullerian agenesis: diagnosis, management, and treatment. Obstet Gynecol. 2013;121(5):1134–7.

21. Roberts CP, Haber MJ, Rock JA. Vaginal creation for mullerian agenesis. Am J Obstet Gynecol. 2001;185(6):1349–52; discussion 1352–3.

22. Edmonds DK, Rose GL, Lipton MG, Quek J. Mayer-Rokitansky-Kuster-Hauser syndrome: a review of 245 consecutive cases managed by a multidisciplinary approach with vaginal dilators. Fertil Steril. 2012;97(3):686–90.

23. Nadarajah S, Quek J, Rose GL, Edmonds DK. Sexual function in women treated with dilators for vaginal agenesis. J Pediatr Adolesc Gynecol. 2005;18(1):39–42.

24. Calcagno M, Pastore M, Bellati F, Plotti F, Maffucci D, Boni T, et al. Early prolapse of a neovagina created with self-dilatation and treated with sacrospinous ligament suspension in a patient with Mayer-Rokitansky-Kuster-Hauser syndrome: a case report. Fertil Steril. 2010;93(1):267.e1–4.

25. Peters 3rd WA, Uhlir JK. Prolapse of a neovagina created by self-dilatation. Obstet Gynecol. 1990;76 (5 Pt 2):904–6.

26. Callens N, De Cuypere G, De Sutter P, Monstrey S, Weyers S, Hoebeke P, et al. An update on surgical and non-surgical treatments for vaginal hypoplasia. Hum Reprod Update. 2014;20(5):775–801.

27. McIndoe A. The treatment of congenital absence and obliterative condition of the vagina. Br J Plast Surg. 1950;2:254–67.

28. Woods J, Alter G, Meland B, Podratz K. Experience with vaginal reconstruction utilizing the modified Singapore flap. Plast Reconstr Surg. 1992;90:270–4.

29. Dhall K. Amnion graft for treatment of congenital absence of the vagina. Br J Obstet Gynaecol. 1984;91(3):279–82.

30. Lin WC, Chang CY, Shen YY, Tsai HD. Use of autologous buccal mucosa for vaginoplasty: a study of eight cases. Hum Reprod. 2003;18(3):604–7.

31. Sharma JB, Gupta N, Mittal S. Creation of neovagina using oxidized cellulose (surgical) as a surgical treatment of vaginal agenesis. Arch Gynecol Obstet. 2007;275(4):231–5.

32. Noguchi S, Nakatsuka M, Sugiyama Y, Chekir C, Kamada Y, Hiramatsu Y. Use of artificial dermis and recombinant basic fibroblast growth factor for creating a neovagina in a patient with Mayer-Rokitansky-Kuster-Hauser syndrome. Hum Reprod. 2004;19(7):1629–32.

33. Panici P, Bellati F, Boni T, Francescangeli F, Frati L, Marchese C. Vaginoplasty using autologous in vitro cultured vaginal tissue in a patient with Mayer von Rokitansky Kuster Hauser syndrome. Human Reprod. 2007;22(7):2025–8.

34. Benedetti Panici P, Maffucci D, Ceccarelli S, Vescarelli E, Perniola G, Muzii L, et al. Autologous in vitro cultured vaginal tissue for vaginoplasty in women with Mayer-Rokitansky-Kuster-Hauser syndrome: anatomic and functional results. J Minim Invasive Gynecol. 2015;22(2):205–11.

35. Grimsby GM, Baker LA. The use of autologous buccal mucosa grafts in vaginal reconstruction. Curr Urol Rep. 2014;15:428.

36. Zhao M, Li P, Li S, Li Q. Use of autologous micromucosa graft for vaginoplasty in vaginal agenesis. Ann Plast Surg. 2009;63:645–9.

37. Davydov SN. Colpopoeisis from the peritoneum of the uterorectal space. Akush Ginekol (Mosk). 1969;45(12):55–7.

38. Fedele L, Frontino G, Restelli E, Ciappina N, Motta F, Bianchi S. Creation of a neovagina by Davydov's laparoscopic modified technique in patients with Rokitansky syndrome. Am J Obstet Gynecol. 2010;202(1):33.e1–6.

39. Labus LD, Djordjevic ML, Stanojevic DS, Bizic MR, Stojanovic BZ, Cavic TM. Rectosigmoid vaginoplasty in patients with vaginal agenesis: sexual and psychosocial outcomes. Sex Health. 2011;8(3):427–30.

40. Williams EA. Congenital absence of the vagina: a simple operation for its relief. J Obstet Gynaecol Br Commonw. 1964;71:511–2.

41. Creatsas G, Deligeoroglou E, Makrakis E, Kontoravdis A, Papadimitriou L. Creation of a neovagina following Williams vaginoplasty and the Creatsas modification in 111 patients with Mayer-Rokitansky-Kuster-Hauser syndrome. Fertil Steril. 2001;76(5):1036–40.

42. Brucker SY, Gegusch M, Zubke W, Rall K, Gauwerky JF, Wallwiener D. Neovagina creation in vaginal agenesis: development of a new laparoscopic Vecchietti-based procedure and optimized instruments in a prospective comparative interventional study in 101 patients. Fertil Steril. 2008; 90(5):1940–52.

43. Fedele L, Bianchi S, Frontino G, Fontana E, Restilli E, Bruni V. The laparoscopic Vecchietti's modified technique in Rokitansky syndrome: anatomic, functional, and sexual long-term results. Am J Obstet Gynecol. 2008;198:377. e1–6.

44. Rall K, Schickner MC, Barresi G, Schonfisch B, Wallwiener M, Wallwiener CW, et al. Laparoscopically assisted neovaginoplasty in vaginal agenesis: a long-term outcome study in 240 patients. J Pediatr Adolesc Gynecol. 2014;27(6):379–85.

45. Raziel A, Friedler S, Gidoni Y, Ben Ami I, Strassburger D, Ron-EI R. Surrogate in vitro fertilization outcome in typical and atypical forms of Mayer-Rokitansky-Kuster-Hauser syndrome. Human Reprod. 2012;27(1):126–30.

46. Brannstrom M, Johannesson L, Bokstrom H, Kvarnstrom N, Molne J, Dahm-Kahler P, et al. Livebirth after uterus transplantation. Lancet. 2014;385(9968):607–16.

Part III

Lateral Anomalies

The Septate Uterus

7

Staci E. Pollack, M. Alexa Clapp,
and Michelle Goldsammler

Incidence

A septate uterus is a type of congenital uterine malformation whereby there is a midline, longitudinal band dividing the uterus either partially (incomplete or subseptate) or completely. This septation may continue caudally, and be associated with a longitudinal vaginal septum. The septate uterus is the most common type of uterine anomaly, with a mean incidence of 35 % amongst all uterine abnormalities, and accounting for ~55 % of uterine malformations when including both septate and arcuate uteri [1]. When looking at the ratio of septate to bicornuate uteri in different patient populations, septate uteri are always more common at a ratio of 4:1, 5:1, and 7:1 in the infertile, general, and recurrent miscarriage populations, respectively [2]. A septate uterus is frequently associated with a complete or partial longitudinal vaginal septum [3],

with 94 % of complete septate uteri associated with a concurrent vaginal septum in one series [4].

The true incidence of a septate uterus is difficult to determine, as the majority of cases go undiagnosed. Most women with a septate uterus will not have any clinical consequences, and therefore, a work-up and evaluation will never be performed. In addition, the criteria for diagnosis are not consistent and all diagnostic testing methods are not equally optimal. The majority of studies are based on women with pregnancy loss and/or infertility, and therefore do not reflect the underlying prevalence in the general population.

The incidence of congenital uterine malformations varies between studies, and has been reported as low as 0.1 % and as high has 12 % [5]. According to a recent systematic review by Chan et al. in 2011, when utilizing optimal tests for diagnosing uterine anomalies (three-dimensional transvaginal sonography, magnetic resonance imaging (MRI), saline infusion vaginal sonohysterography, laparoscopy/laparotomy plus hysteroscopy, or hysterosalpingogram), the overall prevalence of all uterine anomalies was 5.5 % in an unselected population verses 24.5 % in an infertility plus recurrent miscarriage population, and the prevalence of a septate uterus was 2.3 % in an unselected population verses 15.4 % in an infertility plus recurrent miscarriage population [6]. In studies looking at women without infertility or recurrent miscarriage, 5.5–9.8 % were found to have a uterine anomaly, and 2.2–4.3 % were found to specifically have a septate

S.E. Pollack, M.D. (✉)
Obstetrics and Gynecology & Women's Health,Division of Reproductive Endocrinology & Infertility, Montefiore Medical Center, Albert Einstein College of Medicine,
Bronx, NY, USA
e-mail: staci.pollack@einstein.yu.edu

M. Goldsammler • M.A. Clapp, M.D.
Obstetrics Gynecology and Women's Health,
Montefiore Medical Center, Belfer Education Center,
1300 Morris Park Ave, Bronx, NY 10463, USA
e-mail: Mgoldsam@montefiore.org;
mclapp@montefiore.org

© Springer International Publishing Switzerland 2016
S.M. Pfeifer (ed.), *Congenital Müllerian Anomalies*, DOI 10.1007/978-3-319-27231-3_7

uterus, either partial or complete, by three-dimensional transvaginal sonography or saline infusion vaginal sonohysterography, respectively [7, 8]. Furthermore, it is estimated that 1 % of fertile women have a septate uterus [9]. Amongst women seeking treatment for subfertility, 10–15 % will have an intracavitary abnormality [10], and of those women with a diagnosis of unexplained infertility, 1–3.6 % will have a septate uterus [2]. According to the systematic review sited above, utilizing optimal tests, the prevalence of a septate uterus was consistent with prior studies, finding 3 % in an infertility population, and 5.3 % in a recurrent miscarriage population [6].

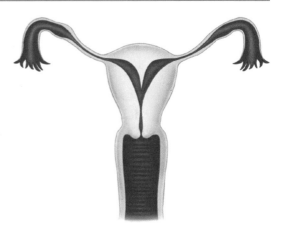

Fig. 7.1 Partial uterine septum: narrow or thin

Etiology

Uterine anomalies are testaments to defects that occur during embryological development, and the septate uterus is no exception. The vast majority of woman with congenital uterine anomalies have normal 46, XX karyotypes, although abnormal karyotypes can be found in 7.7 % of woman with uterine anomalies [11]. To understand the etiology of the septate uterus, it is important to understand normal Müllerian development. Embryonic development of the uterus and surrounding structures takes place between weeks 6 and 16, but can continue as late as week 20. Initially, there are two Müllerian ducts and two Wolffian ducts, both of which are present by week 6. By week 9, the Müllerian ducts have elongated to consist of three segments: (1) the cranial vertical portion which will eventually develop into the fimbriated ends of the Fallopian tubes; (2) the horizontal portion that becomes the isthmus of the Fallopian tubes; and (3) the caudal vertical portion which will migrate to join its contralateral pair to form the uterovaginal primordium (UVP). The UVP will become the uterus, cervix, and upper third of the vagina. The migration of the Fallopian tubes, followed by fusion and internal canalization of the two Müllerian ducts, resulting in two cavities divided by a septum, occurs between weeks 9 and 12 in most cases. This is followed by a period of regression of the partition between the two cavities, thought to be a product of Bcl-2 regulated

apoptosis, usually occurring between week 12 and 16 and resulting in a single cavity [12]. The resorption of the septum is completed by week 20. Thus, normal uterine development involves a complex series of events including Müllerian duct elongation, fusion, canalization, and septal resorption.

A septate uterus results from failure of resorption of the midline partition between the two Müllerian ducts resulting in a fibromuscular septum with a normal external uterine contour. The extent of the septum is variable, from involving the superior aspect of the endometrial cavity (incomplete septum, partial, or subseptate uterus) to a septum that extends the total length of the uterine cavity down to the internal cervical os and including either a cervical septum or complete duplicated cervix (compete septum). A complete or partial longitudinal vaginal septum is found most frequently in concert with a complete septate uterus [3], with 94 % of complete septate uteri associated with a concurrent vaginal septum in one series [4] (Figs. 7.1, 7.2, 7.3, and 7.4).

The current American Society for Reproductive Medicine (ASRM) classification system [13] is based on the classification described by Buttram in 1979 [14] and follows the unidirectional theory of caudal-to-cranial Müllerian duct resorption [13–15]. While this unidirectional theory explains the majority of septate uteri, whereby partial septate uteri contain only the more cephalad portion of the septum, it does not explain the less common anomaly of a complete uterine septum, double cervix, and longitudinal

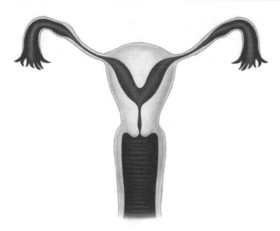

Fig. 7.2 Partial septum: wide or thick

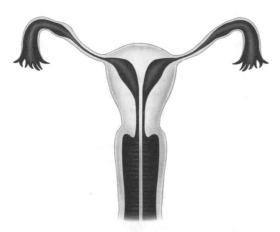

Fig. 7.3 Complete septate uterus with septum extending down through the cervix and associated with a longitudinal vaginal septum

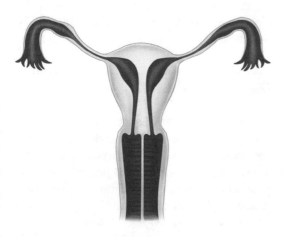

Fig. 7.4 Complete septate uterus with duplicated cervix and longitudinal vaginal septum

vaginal septum first described in 1994 [16]. This less frequent anomaly lends support to the bidirectional/segmental theory of fusion and resorption described by Musset and Muller [17], and championed by Acién in his categorization based on embryological origin [18, 19]. The double cervix is a failure of fusion, occurring between weeks 9 and 12, while the uterine septum is a regression failure during weeks 12–16. Taken together, the complete septate uterus with a double cervix likely results from an insult that occurs around week 12, while a complete septate uterus occurs from a later insult somewhere early between week 12 and 16, and a partial septate uterus ensues from an even later defect as far out as 20 weeks. Additionally, segmental septa also exist, resulting in partitioned uterus with partial communications, and further challenging the unidirectional theory of development [11].

Differential Diagnosis

The differential diagnosis for a septate uterus includes other congenital uterine malformations and is dependent upon which diagnostic test is utilized and which classification system is employed. The European Society of Human Reproduction and Embryology/European Society for Gynaecological Endoscopy (ESHRE/ESGE) classification will overdiagnose septate uteri as compared with the ASRM classification system, diagnosing many uteri as septate that would be considered arcuate or normal by the ASRM classification system [20]. Not only would the ESRE/ESGE system lead to a relative overdiagnosis of septate uteri, but this overdiagnosis may lead to unnecessary treatment without proven benefit [20].

Therefore, the arcuate uterus needs to be distinguished from a true septate uterus. Definitions between the two anomalies are not standardized, and the arcuate uterus has been variably classified as normal, bicornuate, or septate [20, 21]. The arcuate uterus contains a slight residual cranial septum, sometimes with minimal external fundal cavity indentation [21].

Utilizing the ASRM classification system alone is solely subjective. However, several authors have proposed supplementing the ASRM

Table 7.1 AFS Classification system supplemented with proposed additional morphometric criteria [7, 13, 23]

	ASRM Classification	Internal uterine cavity indention (cm)	External uterine contour cleft (cm)
Septate uterus	Class V	≥1.5	<1
Arcuate uterus	Class VI	1–1.5	<1
Bicornuate uterus	Class IV	≥1.5	≥1

classification with additional morphometric criteria [7, 22] (Table 7.1). These additional criteria proposed describe a septate uterus as Class V with an internal uterine cavity indentation ≥1.5 cm and an external uterine contour cleft of <1 cm. Similarly, an arcuate uterus is Class VI with an internal indentation of 1–1.5 cm and an external cleft of <1 cm [7, 20, 22–24]. The indentations are measured using a coronal view on imaging and drawing a horizontal line between the intramural parts of both Fallopian tubes. These strict absolute measurement criteria may not allow for the best classification of all size uteri. Utilizing the ESHRE/ESGE criteria, internal fundal indentations of >50 % of the uterine wall thickness are considered a Class U2 septate uterus, as long as the external cleft is <50 % of the largest wall thickness measured in the sagittal plane [20, 25]. There is no distinct arcuate uterus anomaly within the ESHRE/ESGE classification system.

The most important anomaly that needs to be differentiated from a septate uterus is a bicornuate uterus. Both the septate and the bicornuate uterus have a partitioned cavity. Subsequently, on hysteroscopy the appearance of both the septate and bicornuate uterus is similar. However, the external contour of these two uterine abnormalities is different, and a misdiagnosis can result in complications if a septum resection is performed hysteroscopically on a bicornuate uterus without realizing where the external surface is. The septate uterus has an external counter with a smooth appearance at the fundus, whereas the bicornuate uterus has an external counter with an indented appearance at the fundus that is often described as

heart shaped [26]. Utilizing the ASRM classification system supplemented with distinct morphometric criteria (Table 7.1), the bicornuate uterus is Class IV with an internal indentation of ≥1.5 cm and an external cleft of ≥1 cm [7, 20, 22–24]. Without the morphometric criteria, the distinction between septate and bicornuate uteri was subjective.

It is also important to distinguish between a complete and a partial uterine septum. Resection of a complete uterine septum requires a slightly different surgical technique, which is described below. Patients can also have different variations of complete septate uteri that may include a double cervix and a longitudinal vaginal septum. When two distinct cervices are noted on pelvic examination, the most common diagnosis is uterus didelphys, but one must consider the less common anomaly of a complete uterine septum, double cervix, and longitudinal vaginal septum, first described in 1994. Both of these abnormalities would be treated differently with regard to reproductive outcomes [16]. In addition, it is important to distinguish between a true cervical duplication verses a complete uterine septum through the cervix [27]. If a longitudinal vaginal septum is present, it is commonly resected at the time of uterine septum resection and may even be resected earlier for the indication of dyspareunia or to allow effective tampon use. When a longitudinal vaginal septum is diagnosed in a patient during a basic gynecological well-woman exam, further imaging for any other Müllerian anomalies should be performed.

Diagnosis (Table 7.1)

The diagnosis of a uterine septum, like all uterine anomalies, can be made by utilizing different diagnostic modalities. Diagnostic modalities include both radiologic imaging and surgical procedures. Radiologic modalities include: two-dimensional (2D) and three-dimensional (3D) ultrasound (via transvaginal, transabdominal, or transperineal route), hysterosalpingography (HSG), sonohysterography (SIS), and MRI. According to

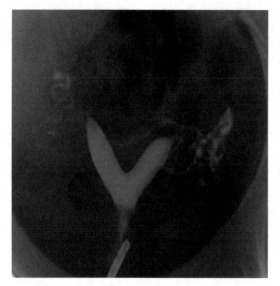

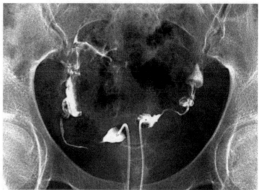

Fig. 7.6 HSG of complete septate uterus. Note the two separate cervical canals and the disparate uterine horns. HSG cannot reliably differentiate complete septate from didelphys uterus (*Image provided by Samantha M. Pfeifer MD*)

Fig. 7.5 HSG of partial septate uterus. The septum depicted here is wide. Note that HSG cannot differentiate between septate and bicornuate uterus (*Image provided by David E Reichman MD*)

a recent systematic review by Chan et al. in 2011, diagnostic modalities may be grouped into optimal tests and suboptimal tests, according to their diagnostic accuracy [6]. Optimal tests include 3D transvaginal ultrasound, MRI, SIS, and laparoscopy or laparotomy plus hysteroscopy or hysterosalpingogram; while suboptimal tests include 2D ultrasound, hysteroscopy alone, HSG, and assessment during Cesarean section [6].

Surgery was historically the gold standard before more advanced imaging techniques were developed. Surgery, specifically simultaneous laparoscopy and hysteroscopy, can aid in the diagnosis of a uterine septum, and enables the provider to treat the uterine malformation at the same time. Hysteroscopy visualizes the intrauterine septum, and laparoscopy visualizes the external counter of the fundus, aiding in the differentiation between a septate and bicornuate uterus. The laparoscopy also enables assessment of the pelvis, including the ovaries and Fallopian tubes. The diagnostic accuracy for the two procedures is 100 % [5]. Surgery, however, is invasive and expensive. With the advent of more advanced imaging modalities, MRI has replaced surgery as the gold standard for the diagnosis of uterine anomalies, such as septums [28].

HSG can assess the uterine cavity and Fallopian tube patency (Figs. 7.5 and 7.6). It cannot, however, assess the external uterine contour and thus has limitations in differentiating between uterine anomalies. The intercornual angle can be determined from an HSG, which will help direct the diagnosis. The angle for a bicornuate uterus is said to be greater than 105° and the angle for a septate uterus is less than 75° [29]. Cases with an angle between 75 and 105° create a diagnostic dilemma, where further diagnostic tools are needed to determine a diagnosis. Unfortunately, accuracy has been cited as only 44 % for an HSG diagnosing different anomalies [29]. Valle and et al. similarly cites the diagnostic accuracy of HSG as 55 % in differentiating a bicornuate from a septate uterus [5]. In addition, a complete septum may be falsely diagnosed as a unicornuate uterus, if the catheter only enters on one side of the septum.

A 2D transvaginal ultrasound can be used as an initial screening test, with its reported sensitivity of up to 90–92 % for uterine anomalies [29]. The sensitivity for diagnosing a septum has been reported as high as 81 % [5]. The ultrasound is best performed during the secretory phase, as this will aid in visualization of the endometrium due to its hyperechoic appearance [30]. A diagnosis of bicornuate uterus is made when the internal indentation is ≥1.5 cm and external contour reveals a fundal cleft of ≥1 cm. Even more sensitive is a 3D ultrasound, which creates a rendering

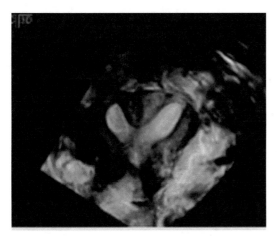

Fig. 7.7 3D US of septate uterus depicted on HSG in Fig. 7.5 (*Image provided by David E Reichman MD*)

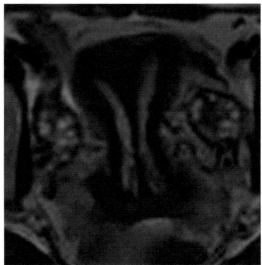

Fig. 7.8 MRI of complete septate uterus. Note the uterine fundus is convex and unified with two separate endometrial cavities. This is the same patient with HSG in Fig. 7.5 (*Image provided by Samantha M. Pfeifer MD*)

image from the typical sagittal and transverse planes (Fig. 7.7). The rendering image provides evaluation of both the internal cavity and the external contour in the coronal plane, thus improving the diagnostic accuracy [29]. A 3D ultrasound can provide a diagnostic accuracy of 92 % for a septum and 100 % for a bicornuate uterus [5]. In addition to having high diagnostic accuracy, the 3D ultrasound is easy to perform, noninvasive, convenient for patients, and can be performed in an office setting [31].

An adjuvant to routine sonography is the SIS, which is best performed during the proliferative phase of the cycle when the endometrium is thin, and involves the introduction of fluid into the cavity to enhance internal delineation. An SIS can be done in either a 2D or a 3D modality [29]. A 3D SIS has improved accuracy and is superior to MRI or office hysteroscopy for classifying uterine anomalies [32]. It is important to note that SIS is a more invasive procedure than 2D or 3D sonography, and except in cases where the endometrial lining is thin, it is unclear if SIS offers any diagnostic advantage over 3D ultrasound [33].

MRI remains the current gold standard for the diagnosis of uterine anomalies for most, with a 100 % sensitivity and accuracy [29] (Fig. 7.8). For distinguishing a bicornuate uterus, MRI uses a greater than 1 cm fundal external cleft, similar to ultrasound morphometric criteria. MRI has advantages of also being able to simultaneously

assess the renal system, which can be effected in many congenital uterine anomalies. While MRI provides an accurate diagnosis, the imaging test is expensive and can be difficult for claustrophobic patients. Berger and et al. concluded that a 3D ultrasound and a 3D SIS provide similar diagnostic accuracy compared to an MRI and do so at decreased cost [29]. Faivre et al. found 3D ultrasound to have improved diagnostic accuracy above MRI [32]. Therefore, 3D ultrasounds may replace MRI as the gold standard for diagnosing uterine anomalies, such as uterine septums [29].

Treatment

Indications

The indications for metroplasty of a septate uterus are controversial, as few have evidence of benefit. Metroplasty may be performed by the transabdominal or hysteroscopic route. However, with advances in the less invasive hysteroscopic techniques, the abdominal approaches have largely been abandoned. The most accepted indication for surgical correction is recurrent pregnancy loss, which usually occurs in the first trimester. Of note, pregnancy loss occurs in only 20–25 % of patients with a septate uterus [5]. Other indications have included infertility or subfertility; however, the strength of this indication is weaker given the fact that a septate uterus does not usually contribute to the etiology of infertility [5]. Observational studies have demonstrated improved spontaneous pregnancy rates after hysteroscopic metroplasty [34], and three observational studies found benefit for removing a uterine septum by hysteroscopic metroplasty in subfertile and infertile women with a uterine septum [35–37].

Patients undergoing assisted reproductive technology (ART) may also undergo resection of a uterine septum prior to their planned treatment. Few quality studies evaluating the benefit of this exist. A retrospective study evaluating pregnancy and live birth rates in women undergoing in vitro fertilization (IVF)/intracytoplasmic sperm injection (ICSI) found lower pregnancy rates, lower live birth rates, and higher miscarriage rates in women with complete septate or partial septate or arcuate uteri, as compared with normal uteri; these differences in reproductive outcomes disappeared after hysteroscopic septum resection [37]. In a historical cohort study of women undergoing IVF, reproductive outcomes were no different between women with normal uterine cavities and women treated with hysteroscopic metroplasty for either a complete uterine septum, incomplete uterine septum, or arcuate uterus [38]. These studies suggest that metroplasty prior to undergoing ART could be indicated in patients with a uterine septum, and that such treatment is not detrimental to reproductive outcomes.

Surgical Adjuvants

Regardless of indication, when surgery is planned, the best timing for the surgery is in the early follicular phase, as the endometrial lining will be thin and therefore aid in surgical visualization. Although combined oral contraceptives and progestins are commonly used preoperatively to thin the lining, Danazol and gonadotropin-releasing hormone (GnRH) agonists have also been used [5, 39].

Various hormonal treatments have been utilized postoperatively to promote endometrial healing and reduce scarring with no proven benefit, although there are no randomized controlled trials evaluating this and the published studies are small and usually retrospective [40]. Nonetheless, postoperative estrogen is often used to induce endometrial growth, followed by a progestin to induce a withdrawal bleed [5]. Of note, complete healing occurs within 8 weeks of hysteroscopic metroplasty [41].

The utilization of intrauterine anti-adhesion agents, stents, Foley catheters, and intrauterine devices (IUDs) were all originally utilized with the intent to prevent adhesion formation. However, although the published literature is relatively poor on this topic, none have been found to be superior to no treatment following hysteroscopic metroplasty and are not routinely used [5]. In addition, the incision of a uterine septum does not usually result in intrauterine adhesion formation, unlike hysteroscopic lysis of synechiae where adhesion reformation is common [5]. In 2010, Tonguc et al. performed a randomized, prospective trial on 100 women who had undergone hysteroscopic metroplasty and were randomized to one of four postoperative treatments: no treatment, daily estradiol + norgestrel (synthetic progestin), copper IUD, or daily estradiol + norgestrel + copper IUD [42]. There was no statistically significant difference in adhesion formation nor pregnancy rates amongst any of the post-surgery treatment regimens although the study was substantially underpowered [42]. One prospective randomized study in 16 patients undergoing hysteroscopic metroplasty evaluated the use of intrauterine auto-crosslinked hyaluronic acid gel administered immediately following incision compared to no therapy [43]. The incidence of postoperative adhesions assessed by hysteroscopy was lower in the gel group compared to controls (12.5 % vs. 37.5 %, respectively, $P<0.05$).

While prophylactic antibiotics are often used, there are no randomized trials examining the use of prophylactic antibiotics in the setting of hysteroscopic metroplasty, nor any randomized trials examining the use of prophylactic antibiotics to reduce infectious morbidity during transcervical intrauterine procedures, and their use is provider preference based [5, 44]. There is one randomized controlled trial looking at prophylactic antibiotics during hysteroscopic procedures, which found no benefit in terms of reducing bacteremia [45]. This taken together with the low risk of infection after metroplasty questions the utility of the use of prophylactic antibiotics to lower the risk of febrile morbidity during hysteroscopic metroplasty [40]. However, it is important to note that no study has looked at subsequent fertility as an outcome after prophylactic antibiotics, and the role of prophylactic antibiotics for this indication is unknown.

Abdominal Procedures

Historically, metroplasty was performed via an abdominal approach using the Jones method or the Tompkins method. Compared to the currently preferred hysteroscopic approach, the abdominal approach had more limitations, including need for laparotomy, greater estimated blood loss, longer hospital stay, prolonged recovery, mandatory cesarean section in succeeding pregnancies, and increased risk of abdominal-pelvic adhesions, which could affect future fertility [5, 39]. The Jones metroplasty involves a wedge resection, which removes a portion of the uterine fundus and the septum [46]. The two uterine halves are then approximated and closed in multiple layers. On the other hand, the Tompkins metroplasty does not remove a portion of the uterine fundus. An incision is made in the anterior–posterior plane, the septum is then removed from each uterine half, and the two halves approximated and closed starting at the base anteriorly and posteriorly [5, 46]. The modified Tompkins metroplasty involves just incising the septum rather than excising it once the uterus is opened as the septal tissue retracts in a similar fashion to the hysteroscopic procedures. To reduce bleeding, diluted vasopressin may be injected into the myometrium or a tourniquet applied around the uterine or uterine and infundibulopelvic vessels. These techniques have been largely replaced by the hysteroscopic techniques described below.

Hysteroscopic Procedures

The hysteroscopic, minimally invasive, approach has since replaced the abdominal approach. This approach offers patients outpatient surgery with shorter recovery time, decreased complication rates, and the possibility of a subsequent vaginal delivery [5, 39]. There are several different hysteroscopic instruments and tools that can be used for a septum resection. The most commonly used are hysteroscopic scissors and electrosurgical instruments, but other techniques include the use of lasers (argon and neodymium:yttrium-aluminum-garnet (Nd:YAG) lasers), vaporizing or bipolar electrodes, and mechanical morcellators [40]. Regardless of tool used, typically, the septum is incised to the level of the myometrium or until bleeding is noted within the tissue, representative of myometrium, and/or the surgeon is able to visualize both tubal ostia within the same panoramic view [40].

Different techniques offer various benefits, but only limited studies have examined superiority of different techniques with regard to reproductive outcomes. Hysteroscopic metroplasty utilizing scissors afforded more pregnancies than when utilizing the resectoscope, according to a study of 81 women by Cararach et al. [47]. Scissors have the disadvantage of being delicate and needing to be changed, adding to the cost, however their use requires minimal dilation and may be done in the outpatient setting. Fedele et al. found no difference between hysteroscopy done with the scissors, the argon laser, or the resectoscope, but this is contradicted by other studies [9].

The simplicity, speed, low cost, and low complication rate lead to electrosurgical procedures being commonly utilized, including the resectoscope [38]. Common electrosurgical instruments include the monopolar resectoscope and the bipolar Versapoint (Gynecare, Ethicon, Somerville, NJ). In a study comparing the resectoscope (knife electrode) and the Versapoint (twizzle-tip electrode) during hysteroscopic metroplasty on 160 women, Colacurci et al. found similar reproductive outcomes between the two groups, including pregnancy rates, abortion rates, gestational age at delivery, and method of delivery [48]. However, patients in the resectoscope group required greater cervical dilation (Hegar size 10 dilator to fit a 26F resectoscope verses often no dilation with the 5 mm Versapoint), had longer operative times (23.4±5.6 vs. 15.7±4.7 min), higher complication rates (total of 7 cases verses 1 case), and greater mean fluid absorption (486.4±169.9 vs. 222.1±104.9 mL) compared to the Versapoint group [48]. A second study by Litta et al. also compared the resectoscope and Versapoint for hysteroscopic metroplasty, with similar findings of equivalent reproductive outcomes but longer operating times and higher complication rates for the resectoscope group [49]. More recent studies found that utilizing the resectoscope with a 0° semicircular loop, as opposed to the 90° Collin's loop, is more manageable and faster [40].

Laser techniques have also been used for hysteroscopic metroplasty but are less widely used. The fiberoptic Nd:YAG laser offers the ability to perform surgery under local anesthesia in the office setting and with minimal cervical dilation to 6.5 mm, but its use is limited by its high cost [50, 51]. While the Nd:YAG laser offers as much as a 98 % success rate according to a study by Yang et al. on 46 patients, the argon laser was found to be less effective than the scissors in a study by Candiani et al. on 21 patients [50, 51].

Historically, the hysteroscopic metroplasty always required concurrent laparoscopy to avoid uterine perforation, and to distinguish between a septate and bicornuate uterus. Today, if the diagnosis of a uterine septum is not confirmed and there is still a possibility of a bicornuate uterus, a simultaneous laparoscopy can be performed with the hysteroscopy to help distinguish between the two diagnoses. A concurrent laparoscopy can also be helpful during a hysteroscopic metroplasty to monitor the depth of the resection in order to minimize the risk of uterine perforation.

The hysteroscope light can also be visualized laparoscopically when the resection is closer to the outer myometrium and serosa [39]. Additionally, the laparoscopy can diagnosis any other pelvic pathology that could be contributing to the infertility etiology. However, simultaneous transabdominal ultrasound monitoring may be preferred to the laparoscopic observation in those in whom the diagnosis is known, and there is no indication for evaluation of the pelvis at the time of hysteroscopic metroplasty. Simultaneous ultrasound has the advantage of being less invasive than laparoscopic observation and provides better ability to gauge the septal division depth in relation to the outer contour of the uterus thereby reducing the risk of uterine perforation [5]. Bettocchi et al. have suggested that by adopting three criteria, a safe, outpatient hysteroscopic metroplasty can distinguish between a septate and bicornuate uterus, without laparoscopic or ultrasound guidance, in approximately 80 % of cases; these three criteria are the presence of vascularized tissue, sensitive innervation, and the appearance of tissue at the site of supposed septum incision [40, 52].

A partial uterine septum is the most common type of uterine septum. When a complete uterine septum or a complete uterine septum with duplicated cervix is present, a different hysteroscopic technique is required for treatment. Typically, a perforation is made in the complete septum, and then the septum is resected in a similar fashion to the partial septum, which was described above. There have been several different instruments described, such as a plastic dilator, Foley catheter, and metal dilator, that can aid the surgeon in finding a location to safely perform the primary septum perforation [53].

Complete septate uteri with cervical duplication also require special attention. Wang et al. performed hysteroscopic metroplasty on 25 women with complete septate uteri with cervical duplication, all who had concurrent laparoscopy and transabdominal ultrasound. A Hank dilator was inserted into one cervix and the 27F hysteroscopic resectoscope (with knife cutting or wire loop electrode) was inserted into the other cervix,

Fig. 7.9 HSG showing complete resection of a septum in complete septate uterus. *Arrows* point to the right and left cervical canals: the HSG cannula in the left cervical canal, the right cervical canal is filling retrograde from the common uterine cavity. Note the fundus of the endometrial cavity is unified and smooth *(Image provided by Samantha M. Pfeifer MD)*

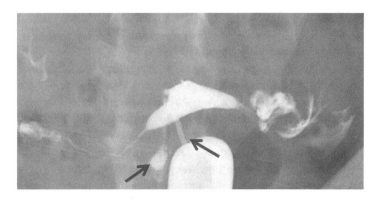

with the Hank dilator serving as a visual marker when the perforation was made in the septum just above the internal os [54]. The Hank dilator also prevented leakage of the distension media through the second cervix [54]. There were no complications and 68.2 % of the cases had no residual septum [54]. Yang et al. compared dilator-guided and light-guided hysteroscopic resections of five complete uterine septums with cervical duplications, concluding that the light-guided instrument was superior in guiding location for the initial septum perforation [55]. Once the septum is resected, the uterine cavity should look normal, with the cervical duplication preserved. Following the procedure it is reasonable to confirm the septum has been satisfactorily resected using saline ultrasound, 3D US, HSG, or hysteroscopy (Fig. 7.9).

In the studies mentioned above, the portion of the septum creating the cervical duplication was preserved. This seems to be the consensus in the literature with the idea to protect the cervical integrity and avoid cervical incompetence in subsequent pregnancies [53–55]. In some situations, the complete uterine septum with duplicated cervix occurs in conjunction with a longitudinal vaginal septum. It is unclear whether this is considered a subset of the complete uterine septum classification or an anomaly that falls into a separate class. If this uncommon anomaly is diagnosed, resection of the vaginal septum can be performed at the same time as the hysteroscopy [53].

Complications

The abdominal metroplasty carries with it a longer operative time and a lengthier postoperative recovery period. Added complications of abdominal metroplasty include risks of bleeding with potential blood transfusion, infection with potential antibiotic therapy, postoperative adhesions that may cause infertility, intrauterine synechiae, full myometrial thickness scar rupture during subsequent pregnancy, and the need for cesarean section in subsequent pregnancy [5, 40].

The minimally invasive approach of a hysteroscopic metroplasty affords less morbidity, but complications can still occur with the minimally invasive route. The overall rate of intra- and postoperative complications is reported to be 1.7 %, according to a systematic review by Nouri et al. in 2010 [56]. These complications are similar to any surgical procedure, including bleeding, infection, and injury to surrounding structures. Intraoperative complications include endocervical or intracavitary injury, such as the creation of false paths, uterine perforation, uterine bleeding, fluid overload, allergic reactions to distending media (such as Dextran 70), and general anesthesia risks [40]. Patients undergoing a hysteroscopic procedure should be aware of the possible need for a laparoscopy or laparotomy if a uterine perforation occurs, in order to evaluate and repair any intra-abdominal injury, such as a bowel injury. As noted above, a conjoint laparoscopy or intraoperative ultrasound monitoring could help decrease the risk of uterine perforation. Volume overload can lead to electrolyte abnormalities and cerebral edema. The total allowable fluid deficit depends on the type of fluids used for the hysteroscopy, which is dependent upon whether monopolar or bipolar instruments are utilized, and an accurate fluid management system greatly aids in monitoring fluid deficits.

Uterine rupture is a rare, late complication of hysteroscopic metroplasty. In a 2005 retrospective literature review, Sentilhes et al. reported only 18 uterine ruptures during subsequent pregnancies following any operative hysteroscopy, and 16 of these had metroplasties [57, 58]. Of note, uterine perforation and/or the use of monopolar cautery increased the risk of subsequent uterine rupture [57, 58]. In a 2013 review and meta-analysis, Valle and Ekpo confirmed 18 reported cases of uterine rupture following hysteroscopic metroplasty [5]. Again of note, during each case of uterine rupture in the literature, there was a hysteroscopic surgical complication recorded, including uterine perforation, excessive septal excision, and excessive use of electrosurgical or laser energy [5].

The risk of intrauterine synechiae after hysteroscopic metroplasty appears to be low [5, 39]. Uterine septal width and surface area have been noted to be predictors of abnormal cavities postoperatively, but this finding is not uniformly noted [45]. Lastly, the need for reoperation after hysteroscopic metroplasty appears to be low, ranging from 0 to 23 %, and being 6 % in a pooled analysis from a systematic literature review [56].

Postoperative Uterine Cavity Evaluation

Postoperatively, the cavity typically is reexamined to evaluate for any residual septum, adhesions, or other anatomic abnormalities. This can be done with imaging or a diagnostic hysteroscopy. A prospective study by Fedele et al. in 1996 compared the reproductive outcomes in patients with a residual septum of between 0.5 and 1 cm to that of a group with no residual septum or a

septum of <0.5 cm. There was no statistically significant difference in reproductive outcomes between the two groups, although the study was underpowered with only 17 patients in the residual septum of 0.5–1 cm arm and 51 patients in the group with no residual septum or septum of <0.5 cm [59].

Impact on Fertility and Reproduction

The presence of a uterine septum increases the risk of a miscarriage; however, many women with a septate uterus have uneventful reproductive function. Only about 20–25 % of patients with a septate uterus experience recurrent miscarriage, typically occurring in the late first and early second trimesters [5]. While the majority of women with septate uteri have successful pregnancies, the septate uterus is the anomaly most frequently associated with pregnancy wastage. Patients with uterine anomalies are at increased risk for obstetrical complications, including malpresentation, preterm labor and birth, premature rupture of membranes, cesarean section, low birth weight, retained placenta, and higher perinatal mortality rates [5, 60]. While a uterine factor can contribute to a patient's presentation of infertility, a uterine septum is not believed to cause infertility.

There have been numerous studies examining the reproductive outcomes in patients after metroplasty. Overall, the literature supports the conclusion that the spontaneous abortion rate is decreased in patients who have undergone surgical correction of a uterine septum [39, 60–62]. A meta-analysis by Venetis et al. in 2014 reported a decreased rate of spontaneous abortion in patients post-hysteroscopic metroplasty (RR 0.37, 95 % CI 0.25–0.55), but did not find any benefit in the likelihood of achieving a pregnancy [60]. A retrospective study from India in 2014 by Gundabattula et al. showed a statistically significant decreased miscarriage rate, increased term delivery rate, increased live birth rate, and increased take home baby rate in the post-resection pregnancies [61]. A retrospective study from Israel by Freud et al. in 2014 examined the reproductive outcomes before and after hysteroscopic metroplasty in 28 patients and showed improved reproductive outcomes in women who have a history of prior spontaneous miscarriage. After the septum resection, the authors noted lower rates of spontaneous miscarriage (12.5 % vs. 63.6 % $p<0.001$), increased mean gestational age at birth (38.47 ± 1.71 weeks vs. 33.73 ± 6.27, $p<0.05$), increased neonatal birth weights (3202.59 ± 630.21 g vs. 2520 ± 764.45, $p<0.05$), and lower risk of preterm delivery (OR = 0.073, 95 % CI 0.16–0.327, $p<0.01$) [62]. Homer et al. in 2000 found lower preterm delivery rates after hysteroscopic metroplasty (6 % vs. 9 %) [39]. While the majority of the studies support the utility of metroplasty in patients with recurrent miscarriages, there are no randomized controlled trials comparing hysteroscopic metroplasty to no intervention, thus limiting the data interpretation [63].

The literature is less clear on the value of metroplasty in treating infertility. While a uterine septum is not felt to cause infertility, metroplasty in women who have infertility appears to improve pregnancy rates. According to a systematic review by Nouri et al. in 2010, hysteroscopic metroplasty is an effective treatment for women with a septate uterus and a history of infertility, resulting in a 60 % pregnancy rate and 45 % live birth rate [56]. A retrospective study by Tehraninejad et al. in 2013 analyzed 203 patients, the majority being infertility patients, who underwent a septum resection. The spontaneous miscarriage rate decreased from 20.2 to 4.9 % after metroplasty ($p<0.0001$), and the rate of term delivery increased from 2.5 to 33.5 % ($p<0.0001$) [64]. A retrospective matched-control study by Tomaževič et al. in 2010 examined women before and after septum resection that were also undergoing ART treatments, with both IVF and ICSI cycles. The rates of pregnancy, live birth, and spontaneous abortion were all improved after metroplasty [37]. These studies suggest that infertility may be another indication for septum resection, besides a history of recurrent pregnancy losses, especially in those women who are planning to proceed with ART.

Conclusions

The septate uterus is the most common of all the uterine anomalies. It is associated with recurrent miscarriage and adverse pregnancy outcomes, including preterm delivery. The role of the septate uterus in infertility is controversial. The best modalities for diagnosing a septate uterus include a 3D ultrasound, with or without saline infusion, and an MRI. Hysteroscopic metroplasty improves reproductive outcomes in women with recurrent miscarriage, and is a simple, well-tolerated procedure with a low complication rate.

References

1. Grimbizis GF, Camus M, Tarlatzis BC, Bontis JN, Devroey P. Clinical implications of uterine malformations and hysteroscopic treatment results. Hum Reprod Update. 2001;7(2):161–74.
2. Saravelos SH, Cocksedge KA, Li TC. Prevalence and diagnosis of congenital uterine anomalies in women with reproductive failure: a critical appraisal. Hum Reprod Update. 2008;14:415–29. doi:10.1093/humupd/dmn018; PMID: 18539641.
3. Haddad B, Louis-Sylvestre C, Poitout P, Paniel BJ. Longitudinal vaginal septum: a retrospective study of 202 cases. Eur J Obstet Gynecol Reprod Biol. 1997;74:197–9.
4. Heinonen PK. Complete septate uterus with longitudinal vaginal septum. Fertil Steril. 2006;85:700–5.
5. Valle RF, Ekpo GE. Hysteroscopic metroplasty for the septate uterus: review and meta-analysis. J Minim Invasive Gynecol. 2013;20:22–42.
6. Chan YY, Jayaprakasan K, Zamora J, Thornton JG, Raine-Fenning N, Coomarasamy A. The prevalence of congenital uterine anomalies in unselected and high-risk populations: a systematic review. Hum Reprod Update. 2011;17(6):761–71.
7. Woelfer B, Salim R, Banerjee S, Elson J, Regan L, Jurkovic D. Reproductive outcomes in women with congenital uterine anomalies detected by three-dimensional ultrasound screening. Obstet Gynecol. 2001;98(6):1099–103.
8. Dreisler E, Stampe Sørensen S. Müllerian duct anomalies diagnosed by saline contrast sonohysterography: prevalence in a general population. Fertil Steril. 2014;102(2):525–9. doi:10.1016/j.fertnstert.2014.04.043. Epub 2014 May 27.
9. Fedele L, Bianchi S, Frontino G. Septums and synechiae: approaches to surgical correction. Clin Obstet Gynecol. 2006;49:767–88.
10. Wallach EE. The uterine factor in infertility. Fertil Steril. 1972;23(2):138–58. PMID: 4551503.

11. Lin PC, Bhatnagar KP, Nettleton GS, et al. Female genital anomalies affecting reproduction. Fertil Steril. 2002;78(5):899–915.
12. Lee DM, Osathanondh R, Yeh J. Localization of Bcl-2 in the human fetal Müllerian tract. Fertil Steril. 1998;70:135–40.
13. American Fertility Society. Classification of adnexal adhesions, distal tubal occlusion, tubal occlusion secondary to tubal ligation, tubal pregnancies, Mullerian anomalies, and intrauterine adhesions. Fertil Steril. 1988;49:944–55.
14. Buttram VC, Gibbons WE. Müllerian anomalies: a proposed classification. (An analysis of 144 cases). Fertil Steril. 1979;32(1):40–6.
15. Crosby WM, Hill EC. Embryology of the Mullerian duct system. A review of present-day theory. Obstet Gynecol. 1962;20:507–15.
16. McBean JH, Brumsted JR. Septate uterus with cervical duplication: a rare malformation. Fertil Steril. 1994;62(2):415–7.
17. Musset R, Muller T, Netter A, Solal E, Vinourd JC, Gillet JV. Etat du haut appareil urinaire chez les porteuses de malformations uterines, etude de 133 observations. Presse Med. 1967;75:1331–6.
18. Acién P, et al. Embryological observations on the female genital tract. Hum Reprod. 1992;7:437–45.
19. Acién P, et al. Complex malformations of the female genital tract. New types and revision of classification. Hum Reprod. 2004;19:2377–84.
20. Ludwin A, Ludwin I. Comparison of the ESHRE-ESGE and ASRM classifications of Mullerian duct anomalies in everyday practice. Hum Reprod. 2015;30:569–80.
21. Rackow BW, Arici A. Reproductive performance of women with Müllerian anomalies. Curr Opin Obstet Gynecol. 2007;19(3):229–37.
22. Ludwin A, Ludwin I, Banas T, Knafel A, Miedzyblocki M, Basta A. Diagnostic accuracy of sonohysterography, hysterosalpingography and diagnostic hysteroscopy in diagnosis of arcuate, septate and bicornuate uterus. J Obstet Gynaecol Res. 2011;37:178–86.
23. Salim R, Woelfer B, Backos M, Regan L, Jurkovic D. Reproducibility of three dimensional ultrasound diagnosis of congenital uterine anomalies. Ultrasound Obstet Gynecol. 2003;21:578–82.
24. Bermejo C, Ten Martınez P, Cantarero R, Diaz D, Perez Pedregosa J, Barron E, Labrador E, Ruiz López L. Three-dimensional ultrasound in the diagnosis of Mullerian duct anomalies and concordance with magnetic resonance imaging. Ultrasound Obstet Gynecol. 2010;35:593–601.
25. Grimbizis GF, Gordts S, Di Spiezio Sardo A, Brucker S, De Angelis C, Gergolet M, Li TC, Tanos V, Brölmann H, Gianaroli L, et al. The ESHRE/ESGE consensus on the classification of female genital tract congenital anomalies. Hum Reprod. 2013;28: 2032–44.
26. Breech LL, Laufer MR. Müllerian anomalies. Obstet Gynecol Clin N Am. 2009;36:47–68.
27. Ludwin A, Ludwin I, Pityński K, Banas T, Jach R. Differentiating between a double cervix or cervical duplication and a complete septate uterus with longitudinal vaginal septum. Taiwan J Obstet Gynecol. 2013;52(2):308–10.
28. Pellerito JS, McCarthy SM, Doyle MB, et al. Diagnosis of uterine anomalies: relative accuracy of MR imaging, endovaginal sonography, and hysterosalpingography. Radiology. 1992;183(3): 795–800.
29. Berger A, Batzer F, Lev-Toaff A, Berry-Roberts C. Diagnostic imaging modalities for Mullerian anomalies: the case for a new gold standard. J Minim Invasive Gynecol. 2014;21:335–45.
30. Nicolini U, Bellotti M, Bonazzi B, et al. Can ultrasound be used to screen uterine malformations? Fertil Steril. 1987;47(1):89–93.
31. Ghi T, Casadio P, Kuleva M, et al. Accuracy of three-dimensional ultrasound in diagnosis and classification of congenital uterine anomalies. Fertil Steril. 2009;92(2):808–13.
32. Faivre E, Fernandez H, Deffieux X, Gervaise A, Frydman R, Levaillant JM. Accuracy of three-dimensional ultrasonography in differential diagnosis of septate and bicornuate uterus compared with office hysteroscopy and pelvic magnetic resonance imaging. J Minim Invasive Gynecol. 2012;19(1):101–6.
33. Ludwin A, Pityński K, Ludwin I, Banas T, Knafel A. Two- and three dimensional ultrasonography and sonohysterography versus hysteroscopy with laparoscopy in the differential diagnosis of septate, bicornuate, and arcuate uteri. J Minim Invasive Gynecol. 2013;20(1):90–9.
34. Taylor E, Gomel V. The uterus and fertility. Fertil Steril. 2008;89(1):1–15.
35. Mollo A, de Franciscis P, Colacurci N, Cobellis L, Perino A, Venezia R, et al. Hysteroscopic resection of the septum improves the pregnancy rate of women with unexplained infertility: a prospective controlled trial. Fertil Steril. 2009;91:2628–31.
36. Shokeir T, Abdelshaheed M, El-Shafei M, Sherif L, Badawy A. Determinants of fertility and reproductive success after hysteroscopic septoplasty for women with unexplained primary infertility: a prospective analysis of 88 cases. Eur J Obstet Gynecol Reprod Biol. 2011;155:54–7.
37. Tomaževič T, Ban-Frangež H, Virant-Klun I, Verdenik I, Požlep B, Vrtačnik-Bokal E. Septate, subseptate and arcuate uterus decrease pregnancy and live birth rates in IVF/ICSI. Reprod Biomed Online. 2010;21(5): 700–5.
38. Abuzeid M, Ghourab G, Abuzeid O, Mitwally M, Ashraf M, Diamond M. Reproductive outcome after IVF following hysteroscopic division of incomplete uterine septum/arcuate uterine anomaly in women with primary infertility. Facts Views Vis Obgyn. 2014;6(4):194–202.
39. Homer HA, Li TC, Cooke ID. The septate uterus: a review of management and reproductive outcome. Fertil Steril. 2000;73(1):1–14.

40. Paradisi R, Barzanti R, Fabbri R. The techniques and outcomes of hysteroscopic metroplasty. Curr Opin Obstet Gynecol. 2014;26(4):295–301.

41. Candiani GB, Vercellini P, Fedele L, Carinelli SG, Merlo D, Arcaini L. Repair of the uterine cavity after hysteroscopic septal incision. Fertil Steril. 1990;54(6): 991–4.

42. Tonguc EA, Var T, Yilmaz N, Batioglu S. Intrauterine device or estrogen treatment after hysteroscopic uterine septum resection. Int J Gynecol Obstet. 2010;109: 226–9.

43. Guida M, Acunzo G, Di Spiezio Sardo A, Bifulco G, Piccoli R, Pellicano M, et al. Effectiveness of auto-crosslinked hyaluronic acid gel in the prevention of intrauterine adhesions after hysteroscopic surgery: a prospective, randomized, controlled study. Hum Reprod. 2004;19:1461–4.

44. Thinkhamrop J, Laopaiboon M, Lumbiganon P. Prophylactic antibiotics for transcervical intrauterine procedures. Cochrane Database Syst Rev. 2013;(5): CD005637.

45. Bhattacharya S, Parkin DE, Reid TM, et al. A prospective randomised study of the effects of prophylactic antibiotics on the incidence of bacteraemia following hysteroscopic surgery. Eur J Obstet Gynecol Reprod Biol. 1995;63:37–40.

46. Damewood MD, Rock JA. Chapter 19: Uterine reconstructive surgery. In: Hunt RB, editor. Text and atlas of female infertility surgery. 3rd ed. St. Louis: Mosby; 1999. p. 274–8.

47. Cararach M, Penella J, Ubeda A, Labastida R. Hysteroscopic incision of the septate uterus: scissors versus resectoscope. Hum Reprod. 1994;9(1):87–9.

48. Colacurci N, Franciscis PD, Mollo A, Litta P, Perino A, Cobellis L, et al. Small diameter hysteroscopy with Versapoint versus resectoscopy with a unipolar knife for the treatment of septate uterus: a prospective randomized study. J Minim Invasive Gynecol. 2007; 14:622–7.

49. Litta P, Spiller E, Saccardi C, Ambrosini G, Caserta D, Cosmi E. Resectoscope or Versapoint for hysteroscopic metroplasty. Int J Gynecol Obstet. 2008;101: 39–42.

50. Yang J, Yin TU, Xu WM, Xia LG, Li AB, Hu J. Reproductive outcome of septate uterus after hysteroscopic treatment with neodymium:YAG laser. Photomed Laser Surg. 2006;24:625–9.

51. Candiani GB, Vercellini P, Fedele L, Garsia S, Brioschi D, Villa L. Argon laser versus microscissors for hysteroscopic incision of uterine septa. Am J Obstet Gynecol. 1991;164(1 Pt 1):87–90.

52. Bettocchi S, Ceci O, Nappi L, Pontrelli G, Pinto L, Vicino M. Office hysteroscopic metroplasty: three "diagnostic criteria" to differentiate between septate and bicornuate uteri. J Minim Invasive Gynecol. 2007;14(3):324–8.

53. Patton PE, Novy MJ, Lee DM, Hickok LR. The diagnosis and reproductive outcomes after surgical treatment of the complete septate uterus, duplicated cervix and vaginal septum. Am J Obstet Gynecol. 2004; 190:1669–78.

54. Wang JH, Xu KH, Lin J, Chen XZ. Hysteroscopic septum resection of complete septate uterus with cervical duplication, sparing the double cervix in patients with recurrent spontaneous abortions or infertility. Fertil Steril. 2009;91:2643–9.

55. Yang JH, Chen MJ, Shih JC, Chen CD, Chen SU, Yang YS. Light-guided hysteroscopic resection of complete septate uterus with preservation of duplicated cervix. J Minim Invasive Gynecol. 2014;21: 940–4.

56. Nouri K, Ott J, Huber JC, Fischer EM, Stoqbauer L, Tempfer CB. Reproductive outcome after hysteroscopic septoplasty in patients with septate uterus—a retrospective cohort study and systematic review of the literature. Reprod Biol Endocrinol. 2010;8:52.

57. Sentilhes L, Sergent F, Roman H, Verspyck E, Marpeau L. Late complications of operative hysteroscopy: predicting patients at risk of uterine rupture during subsequent pregnancy. Eur J Obstet Gynecol Reprod Biol. 2005;120:134–8.

58. Sentilhes L, Sergent F, Berthier A, Catala L, Descamps P, Marpeau L. Uterine rupture following operative hysteroscopy. Gynecol Obstet Fertil. 2006;34(11): 1064–70.

59. Fedele L, Bianchi S, Marchini M, Mezzopane R, Di Nola G, Tozzi L. Residual uterine septum of less than 1cm after hysteroscopic metroplasty does not impair reproductive outcome. Hum Reprod. 1996;11:727–9.

60. Venetis CA, Papadopoulos SP, Campo R, Gordts S, Tarlatzis BC, Grimbizis GF. Clinical implications of congenital uterine anomalies: a meta-analysis of comparative studies. Reprod Biomed Online. 2014;29: 665–83.

61. Gundabattula SR, Joseph E, Marakani LR, Dasari S, Nirmalan PK. Reproductive outcomes after resection of intrauterine septum. J Obstet Gynaecol. 2014; 34:235–7.

62. Freud A, Harlev A, Weintraub AY, Ohana E, Sheiner E. Reproductive outcomes following uterine septum resection. J Matern Fetal Neonatal Med. 2014. doi:10 .3109/14767058.2014.981746.

63. Kowlaik CR, Goddijn M, Emanuel MH, Bongers MY, Spinder T, de Kruif JH, Mol BW, Heineman MJ. Metroplasty verses expectant management for women with recurrent uterus and a septate uterus. Cochrane Database Syst Rev. 2011;(6):CD008576.

64. Tehraninejad ES, Ghaffari F, Jahangiri N, Oroomiechiha M, Akhoond MR, Aziminekoo E. Reproductive outcome following hysteroscopic monopolar metroplasty: an analysis of 203 cases. Int J Fertil Steril. 2013;7: 175–80.

Bicornuate Uterus

8

Lauren Zakarin Safier and Beth W. Rackow

Incidence

The overall incidence of müllerian anomalies in the general population is estimated to be approximately 2 % [1]. Calculating the exact incidence of müllerian anomalies has proven challenging as many women with such anomalies are not diagnosed, especially if asymptomatic. A critical analysis of studies utilizing optimal techniques to diagnose uterine anomalies, specifically hysteroscopy with or without laparoscopy, sonohysterography and three-dimensional ultrasonography, determined that the prevalence of congenital uterine anomalies is approximately 6.7 % in the general population, 7.3 % in the infertile population, and 16.7 % in the recurrent pregnancy loss population [2].

Congenital uterine anomalies occur due to agenesis and hypoplastic defects, lateral fusion defects, and vertical fusion defects of the müllerian ducts. This chapter focuses on the bicornuate uterus, a type of lateral fusion defect. The bicornuate uterus results from incomplete fusion of the müllerian ducts at the level of the fundus, leading to a fundal cleft and a divided endometrial cavity. The bicornuate uterus accounts for 10–25 % of uterine anomalies [3, 4].

Etiology

The female reproductive tract is formed by a series of events, and any derailment can result in a wide array of uterine and vaginal anomalies. Early in embryologic development, both the wolffian (mesonephric) and müllerian (paramesonephric) ducts are present. While genetic sex is determined at the time of fertilization, male or female phenotype is not defined until after the sixth week of development. The paired müllerian ducts arise from coelomic epithelium along the lateral walls of the urogenital ridge, and these solid ducts are present by week 6 of development. In the male fetus, müllerian inhibiting substance (MIS) is produced by the gonads, leading to regression of the müllerian structures. Due to the absence of MIS in the female fetus, the müllerian ducts proliferate while the wolffian ducts regress. Next, the müllerian ducts elongate caudally and cross the wolffian ducts medially, and midline fusion of the ducts forms the primitive uterine structure. By week 10 of development, fusion occurs between the caudal end of the joined müllerian ducts and the urogenital sinus. Once unified, the two solid ducts undergo internal

L. Zakarin Safier, M.D.
Center for Women's Reproductive Care,
1790 Broadway, 4th floor, New York,
NY 10019, USA
e-mail: lz2411@cumc.columbia.edu

B.W. Rackow, M.D. (✉)
Department of Obstetrics and Gynecology,
Columbia University Medical Center, 622 West
168th Street, PH 16-127, New York, NY 10032, USA
e-mail: bwr2113@cumc.columbia.edu

© Springer International Publishing Switzerland 2016
S.M. Pfeifer (ed.), *Congenital Müllerian Anomalies*, DOI 10.1007/978-3-319-27231-3_8

canalization, resulting in two lumens separated by a midline septum, and the septum typically resorbs in a caudal to cephalad direction. Development of the female reproductive tract is completed by 20 weeks of gestation.

A bicornuate uterus results from incomplete lateral fusion of the two müllerian ducts, leading to varying degrees of separation between the two uterine cavities. Thus, a bicornuate uterus consists of two symmetric cornua separated by a midline fundal myometrial cleft and a myometrial division between the cavities that can have varying degrees of length. Within the bicornuate uterine structure, the endometrial cavities can be completely separate or partially communicating at the level of the uterine isthmus. In its mildest form, a slight midline division of the uterine cavity corresponds with a fundal indentation measuring 1 cm or greater. This fundal concavity measurement is utilized to differentiate a bicornuate uterus from a septate uterus, which has no fundal indentation or an indentation of less than 1 cm [5–7]. The intervening fundal cleft of the complete bicornuate uterus can extend to the internal cervical os and creates two separate endometrial cavities. In contrast, the cleft of a partial bicornuate uterus is of variable length and does not extend to the internal os, thus a portion of the endometrial cavity is unified. In addition to variation in length of the midline fundal cleft and the endometrial cavity configuration, bicornuate uteri may have a single cervix (bicornuate unicollis) or a duplicated cervix (bicornuate bicollis) [8]. Several variations of the bicornuate uterus have been described in the literature (Fig. 8.1).

With bicornuate uteri, the variations in the myometrial cleft, endometrial cavity configuration, number of cervices, and other associated anomalies can complicate the presentation and diagnosis. One-fourth of females with bicornuate uteri may also have a longitudinal vaginal septum, and this finding may cause a bicornuate uterus to be misclassified as a uterus didelphys or a complete septate uterus [3]. Transverse vaginal septae, imperforate hymens, and obstructing longitudinal vaginal septae have also been reported with a bicornuate uterus. Furthermore, since the müllerian system and urinary system undergo embryologic development at the same time, renal, ureteral, and other urinary tract anomalies may also be associated with bicornuate uteri as well as with other uterine anomalies [9].

Differential Diagnosis

A female with a uterine anomaly can present with various obstetric or gynecologic issues related to the uterine configuration or associated anomalies. However, many females with a uterine anomaly are asymptomatic, and thus are never diagnosed or are only diagnosed during pregnancy. Obstetrical complications that may lead to detailed uterine evaluation and the diagnosis of a uterine anomaly include recurrent pregnancy loss during the first and second trimester, preterm labor, and malpresentation [10]. Possible gynecologic presentations of a uterine anomaly include dysmenorrhea, abnormal uterine bleeding, and difficulties with an intrauterine device (IUD) including expulsion of an IUD or pregnancy with an IUD in place [11]. Furthermore, a nonobstructing longitudinal vaginal septum associated with a uterine anomaly may present due to difficulty with tampon insertion, bleeding around a tampon (two tampons are needed) or dyspareunia [5]. Lastly, an obstructing longitudinal vaginal septum commonly presents shortly after menarche with cyclic or acyclic pelvic pain secondary to hematometra, hematocolpos, or endometriosis as a result of retrograde menstruation [8]. Rarely, females may present with symptoms of infection such as fever, lower abdominal pain, or foul smelling discharge secondary to a microperforation in the obstructing vaginal septum [7].

When evaluating a female with any of these specific obstetric or gynecologic complaints, a thorough history and physical exam as well as the use of imaging modalities helps provide important clues in the diagnosis of a bicornuate uterus. In the setting of imaging that identifies a partial separation of the endometrial cavity, the differential diagnosis includes a partial bicornuate uterus, partial septate uterus, and arcuate uterus. If the imaging demonstrates two separate endometrial cavities, the differential diagnosis includes a

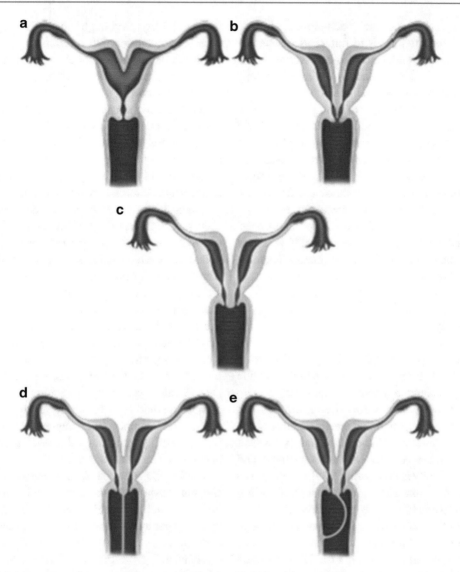

Fig. 8.1 Images of several types of bicornuate uteri. (**a**) Partial bicornuate unicollis, (**b**) complete bicornuate unicollis, (**c**) complete bicornuate bicollis, (**d**) complete bicornuate bicollis with nonobstructing longitudinal vaginal septum, (**e**) complete bicornuate bicollis with obstructing longitudinal vaginal septum

complete bicornuate uterus, complete septate uterus, and didelphys uterus. If cervical duplication is appreciated, this anomaly can be seen with bicornuate, septate, didelphys, and normal uteri. Lastly, a nonobstructing or obstructing longitudinal vaginal septum can occur with bicornuate, septate, didelphys, and normal uteri. Therefore, detailed evaluation of pelvic anatomy is essential to formulate a differential diagnosis and make the proper diagnosis.

Diagnosis

Clinical history and physical examination are the first steps in evaluation of women with a known or possible uterine anomaly. As previously mentioned, a range of obstetric and gynecologic "symptoms" may raise suspicion for a uterine anomaly, but many women with uterine anomalies are asymptomatic. Furthermore, identification of a vaginal or cervical anomaly on physical examination often leads to further assessment of pelvic anatomy and may discover a uterine anomaly. Although surgical evaluation with laparoscopy and hysteroscopy has traditionally been the gold standard for evaluation of complex müllerian anomalies [5], with readily available diagnostic imaging, surgery is rarely necessary for diagnostic purposes. Imaging such as two-dimensional (2D) ultrasound, three-dimensional (3D) ultrasound, and magnetic resonance imaging (MRI) offers a noninvasive and accurate means for evaluating bicornuate uteri and other müllerian anomalies. It is essential that the imaging modality is able to assess the myometrial and endometrial contours to accurately characterize a uterine anomaly.

Imaging

When evaluating a woman with a possible uterine anomaly, 2D ultrasound is often the initial pelvic imaging technique utilized in the office setting. 2D ultrasound allows for visualization of the uterine structure, including the architecture of the myometrium and endometrium, and assessment of the ovaries. A pattern of low sensitivity and high specificity is noted with 2D ultrasound evaluation of uterine anomalies; although 2D ultrasound may only identify approximately half of the uterine anomalies present, the diagnosis of an anomaly is highly likely to be correct [2]. The addition of saline infusion to a 2D ultrasound (saline infusion sonogram; SIS) provides better visualization of intrauterine pathology such as a polyp, submucosal myoma, uterine septum, or intrauterine adhesions. However, even when combining 2D ultrasound with SIS, it remains difficult to differentiate a bicornuate uterus from other uterine anomalies such as a septate uterus or didelphys uterus. In addition, given the possible anatomic variations of bicornuate uteri, more advanced imaging modalities such as 3D ultrasound and MRI are often needed to better characterize a bicornuate uterus and any possible associated anomalies.

A hysterosalpingogram (HSG) is commonly used for the evaluation of tubal patency in women with infertility. Although an HSG may also detect abnormalities of the uterine cavity, its utility in evaluating the cavity is limited because it only provides a 2D representation of a 3D structure. Furthermore, it cannot reliably differentiate between uterine anomalies as an HSG does not evaluate the external contour of the uterus [2]. For instance, when an HSG identifies a 2 cm indentation in the fundal aspect of the cavity, this finding could be due to a partial bicornuate or a partial septate uterus, and additional imaging that evaluates the myometrium and fundal contour is necessary to make this determination. One retrospective study of 155 infertile women who underwent hysterosalpingography identified 118 women with a normal uterus, 4 with a unicornuate uterus, and 6 with a didelphys uterus. In 22 cases, due to the lack of evaluation of the external contour of the uterus, HSG could not differentiate between arcuate, septate, and bicornuate uteri. After performing 3D ultrasound, the diagnoses for the 22 disputed cases were confirmed [12]. While hysterosalpingography is not the optimal method for diagnosing uterine anomalies, it is a common screening test for women with infertility and may discover previously undiagnosed uterine anomalies [12].

Unlike 2D ultrasound, 3D ultrasound can simultaneously assess the architecture of the uterine cavity, the myometrium, and the fundus. 3D ultrasonography has a very high rate of accuracy in diagnosing uterine anomalies [13, 14]. As demonstrated in Fig. 8.2, the coronal view provided by 3D ultrasound allows for differentiation between anomalies such as bicornuate and septate uteri [15]. One study sought to compare the diagnostic accuracy of hysteroscopy and laparoscopy for uterine anomalies to 2D transvaginal ultrasound (TVS), expert transvaginal ultrasound, 2D ultrasound with SIS, and 3D ultrasound with SIS. Hysteroscopy performed in conjunction with laparoscopy detected 23 arcuate, 60 septate, 22 bicornuate, and 12 normal uteri. In comparison, 3D-SIS showed perfect diagnostic accuracy (100.0 %) in the detection of uterine anomalies, compared with 2D-TVS (77.8 %), expert 2D-TVS (90.6 %), 2D-SIS (94.0 %), and 3D-TVS (97.4 %). In the overall diagnosis of uterine anomalies, all

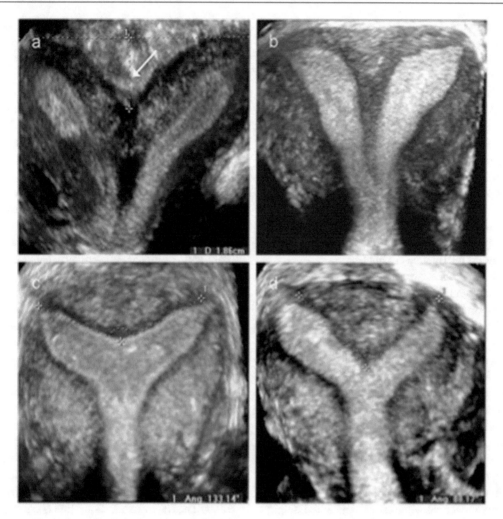

Fig. 8.2 Three-dimensional rendered coronal ultrasound images demonstrating ultrasound criteria for classification of congenital uterine anomalies. (**a**) Bicornuate uterus: two divergent cornua are noted, divided by a sagittal cleft >10 mm (*arrow*). (**b**) Complete septate uterus: a normal external uterine contour is present, and a septum divides the endometrial cavity and extends to the cervix. (**c**) Arcuate uterus: a normal external uterine contour is identified with a concave fundal indentation of the endometrial cavity at an obtuse angle. (**d**) Partial septate uterus: a normal external uterine contour is present, the septum does not extend to the cervix, and the central point of the fundal indentation demonstrates an acute angle. Reprinted with permission from Ghi et al. [15]

imaging methods had significantly better diagnostic capability than 2D-TVS ($p<0.001$), and 3D-SIS was the only method that was significantly better than expert 2D-TVS ($p<0.001$) [16]. With expanded availability of 3D ultrasound and with increased comfort with use of this imaging modality to assess uterine anomalies, 3D ultrasound is an effective tool when evaluating women with uterine anomalies [17].

Similar to 3D ultrasound, MRI can accurately evaluate the architecture of the uterine cavity, the myometrium, and the external uterine fundal contour, allowing for clear differentiation between a lateral fusion anomaly such as a bicornuate uterus or a uterus didelphys, and a resorption anomaly such as a septate uterus [18]. MRI provides detailed delineation of internal and external uterine contours, can differentiate between a myometrial and fibrous uterine division, can differentiate between a septate cervix and a duplicated cervix, and can diagnose vaginal anomalies [3]. The duplicated cervix in the bicornuate bicollis uterus has been described as having an "owl eyes" appearance on MRI [18]. In comparing the diagnostic accuracy of 3D ultrasound and MRI for uterine anomalies, a high degree of concordance between 3D ultrasonography and MRI has been identified (kappa index: 0.878 [95 % CI, 0.775–0.980]). However, discrepancies occurred in the diagnosis of 4 of 65 anomalies; 3D ultrasound misclassified one bicornuate uterus as a didelphys uterus, and three septate uteri as bicornuate uteri [19]. With apparent similarities in diagnostic accuracy for uterine anomalies, other factors must be considered such as cost, availability and quality of equipment, and the experience of the providers interpreting the images.

In addition, for women diagnosed with a müllerian anomaly, investigation of the urinary tract is important to determine if a coexisting abnormality is present. Due to simultaneous embryologic development of the müllerian and urinary systems, a congenital abnormality in one tract should lead to assessment of the other tract. In one study looking at coexisting müllerian and urinary tract malformations, of 38 women with bicornuate uteri, 11 were found to have an associated urinary tract anomaly including unilateral kidney atresia, horseshoe kidney, duplicated ureters, and vesicoureteral reflux [9]. Although renal and urinary tract anomalies occur more commonly in women with unicornuate and didelphys uteri and müllerian agenesis than in those who have bicornuate uteri [7], renal and urinary tract imaging remains an important part of the workup for any female who presents with a müllerian anomaly. Imaging such as renal ultrasound, MRI urogram, CT scan, or intravenous pyelogram may be employed to evaluate the renal and urinary tract; renal ultrasound is the recommended initial test, and further testing can be ordered as indicated [9].

Treatment

Surgical intervention can be utilized for evaluation and treatment of müllerian anomalies. An examination under anesthesia with hysteroscopy and laparoscopy may be performed to evaluate a uterine anomaly in the setting of inadequate imaging, and allows for assessment of the rest of the pelvic structures. Simultaneous evaluation of the external and internal uterine contours can confirm the type of uterine anomaly. For a bicornuate uterus, surgical treatment is rarely indicated. Surgery may be indicated only in the setting of recurrent poor obstetric outcomes such as repetitive late second trimester losses or third trimester preterm deliveries [20]. However, in women with recurrent pregnancy loss or a history of preterm delivery, it is important to rule-out causes other than a structural disorder of the uterus and optimize obstetrical management before considering surgical correction [21].

The Strassman metroplasty, originally described in 1907, is the standard surgical procedure for correction of a complete or partial bicornuate uterus [22]. This procedure should be performed by surgeons with expertise in uterine reconstructive procedures. Prior to performing the Strassman metroplasty procedure, the myometrium is infiltrated with dilute pitressin or a tourniquet is placed around the uterus. Next, a transverse myometrial incision is made from cornua to cornua that starts at least 1 cm away from the insertion of the fallopian tubes into the uterus, and the dissection is carried down to the uterine cavities. The transverse incision line is converted to a vertical suture line that runs from the anterior aspect of the uterus across the midline fundus and down the posterior wall, drawing the lateral halves of the uterus together in the midline. The endometrium and myometrium are reapproximated in several layers. Thus, the uterine cavities are brought together to create one unified cavity [22] (Fig. 8.3). In a series of 22 women who underwent the Strassman metroplasty, 88 % achieved pregnancies and 19 viable infants were born. All pregnancies had unremarkable courses, demonstrating that the post-metroplasty reproductive outcomes of these women were very good [23]. In a prospective analysis of 13 women with bicornuate uteri who underwent abdominal metroplasty according to the Strassman technique, the fetal survival rate increased from 0 % before

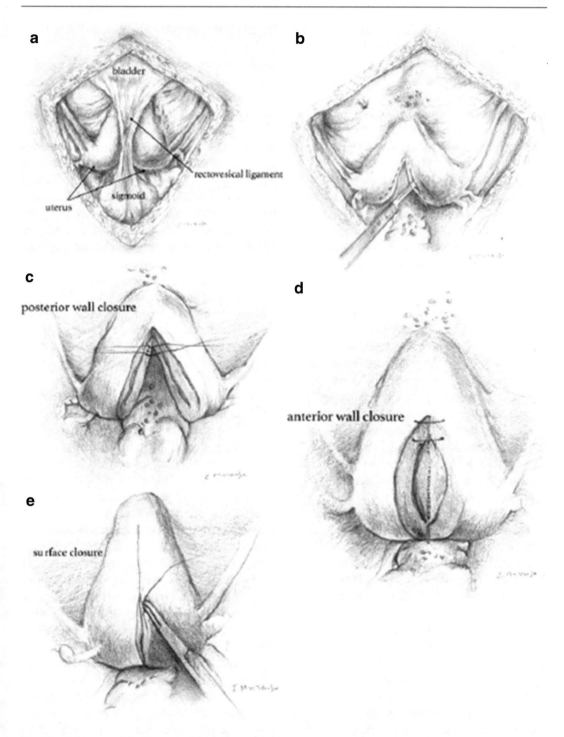

Fig. 8.3 Illustration of the Strassman Metroplasty procedure for unification of a bicornuate uterus: surgical steps. (**a**) Bicornuate uterus. (**b**) Incision from one cornua to the other. (**c**) Posterior endometrial cavity and uterine wall closure. (**d**) Anterior endometrial cavity and uterine wall closure. (**e**) Serosal closure

surgery to 80 % after the operation. No intraoperative and postoperative complications were observed, and no cases of uterine rupture or other intrapartum complications occurred [24]. However, the Strassman metroplasty should be reserved for selected women with bicornuate uteri who have experienced recurrent poor reproductive outcomes such as recurrent pregnancy loss or preterm birth [25].

Historically, the Strassman metroplasty for repair of a bicornuate uterus has been performed by laparotomy, but some surgeons are now performing the procedure with a laparoscopic approach. In one case series involving 26 women with double uterine cavities (22 bicornuate and 4 didelphys uteri) and with a history of recurrent pregnancy loss who underwent laparoscopic Strassman metroplasty, all women were noted to have a unified and acceptable uterine cavity in a second-look operation. Of 10 women with bicornuate uteri who were followed for 1-year post-procedure, 9 women conceived of whom 7 delivered by cesarean section, and 2 had spontaneous abortions, and one woman decided to delay conception [26]. The laparoscopic approach for the Strassman metroplasty appears to be a safe and effective technique for the correction of a bicornuate uterus; however, this approach requires expertise in minimally invasive gynecologic surgery.

Regardless of a laparoscopic or abdominal approach for the Strassman metroplasty, women with bicornuate uteri must be counseled that a scheduled caesarean section is the recommended mode of delivery due to the risk of uterine rupture following a full thickness fundal incision [21]. In addition, to allow for uterine healing after surgery, it is recommended that women postpone attempting conception for at least 3–6 months.

Other malformations associated with bicornuate uteri may warrant surgical intervention, such as obstructing or nonobstructing longitudinal vaginal septae. When present, excision of a vaginal septum is indicated in the setting of obstruction of menstrual flow, and may be indicated for a nonobstructing septum that affects the ability to use tampons, that causes dyspareunia or that prevents adequate cervical screening.

Impact on Fertility/Reproduction

Uterine anomalies do not appear to have a significant impact on fertility and achieving pregnancy, but are associated with an increased risk of recurrent pregnancy loss and obstetrical complications. A systematic review evaluated four groups of women to determine the prevalence of uterine anomalies diagnosed by optimal tests (3D-TVS, laparoscopy, or laparotomy performed with hysteroscopy or HSG, MRI, and SIS). The prevalence of uterine anomalies was 5.5 % in the unselected population, 8.0 % in infertile women, 13.3 % in those with a history of miscarriage, and 24.5 % in those with miscarriage and infertility [27]. Thus, a higher prevalence of uterine anomalies was identified in women with a history of miscarriage or miscarriage plus infertility compared with the unselected population.

In addition to recurrent pregnancy loss, uterine anomalies are associated with other obstetrical complications including preterm delivery, intrauterine growth restriction (IUGR), malpresentation, placental abruption, and retained placenta [28]. These complications are thought to be secondary to decreased uterine muscle mass, abnormal uterine vasculature, and cervical insufficiency [7]. The risk of obstetrical complications also varies with the type of uterine anomaly. A review of reproductive outcomes in women with uterine anomalies determined that women with bicornuate uteri have a spontaneous abortion rate of 36 %, a preterm birth rate of 23 %, a term delivery rate of 40.6 %, and a live birth rate of 55.2 % [4]. Other studies evaluated reproductive outcomes in women with partial vs. complete bicornuate uteri. Although some studies identified a higher frequency of adverse outcomes with partial bicornuate uteri [29, 30], other authors have not found a difference [31]. Furthermore, with a bicornuate uterus, the chance of a successful live birth has been shown to increase with each subsequent pregnancy; this may be related to serial stretching of the myometrium and improved uterine vascularity with each unsuccessful pregnancy [11].

Surgical intervention should be reserved for select women with bicornuate uteri who have experienced poor reproductive outcomes such as recurrent pregnancy loss or preterm birth. Treatment options include the Strassman metroplasty to unify partially or completely divided uterine cavities, and placement of a cervical cerclage for women with a history of preterm dilation and cervical incompetence. In one case–control study, pregnancy outcomes were studied in 40 pregnant women with a bicornuate uterus, of whom 26 had a cervical cerclage placed and 14 did not have a cerclage. In women with a bicornuate uterus and cervical cerclage, delivery occurred at term in 76.2 % and 23.8 % delivered preterm. In contrast, for women with a bicornuate uterus without cervical cerclage, term delivery occurred in 27.3 % and preterm delivery in 72.7 % ($p < 0.05$) of this cohort [32]. Although cervical cerclage may improve fetal survival rates and decrease preterm delivery rates, initial expectant management and appropriate adherence to standard indications for cerclage placement are recommended [10]. Due to the increased obstetrical risk related to uterine anomalies, preconception consultation with a Maternal Fetal Medicine specialist should be encouraged for women with uterine anomalies, and particularly for women with a uterine anomaly and a history of cervical incompetence or other obstetrical complications.

Conclusion

The bicornuate uterus is a type of uterine anomaly that encompasses several anatomic variations including partial or complete divisions between the endometrial cavities, single or duplicated cervices, and associated vaginal anomalies. Women with a bicornuate uterus may be identified at the time of pregnancy, during evaluation of poor obstetrical outcomes or during evaluation of an obstructing or nonobstructing vaginal anomaly, but many women are asymptomatic and remain undiagnosed. Evaluating women with a possible uterine anomaly requires a detailed history and physical examination, and appropriate imaging. It is important to recognize that uterine anomalies with a partially or completely divided endometrial cavity, the bicornuate, septate, and didelphys uteri,

may be mistaken for one another and can have different reproductive implications and management strategies. Furthermore, women with uterine anomalies commonly warrant imaging of the urinary tract to assess for associated anomalies. For women with a bicornuate uterus, conception does not appear to be affected; however, there is an increased risk of obstetrical complications such as recurrent pregnancy loss, preterm labor, IUGR, placental abruption, and cervical incompetence. Surgical intervention with the Strassman metroplasty or cervical cerclage should be considered in select women with a history of recurrent poor obstetrical outcomes.

References

1. Speroff L, Fritz M. Clinical gynecologic endocrinology and infertility. 8th ed. Philadelphia: Lippincott Williams & Wilkins; 2010. p. 1191–220.
2. Saravelos SH, Cocksedge KA, Li TC. Diagnosis of congenital uterine anomalies in women with reproductive failure: a critical appraisal. Hum Reprod Update. 2008;14:415–29.
3. Troiano RN, McCarthy SM. Mullerian duct anomalies: imaging and clinical issues. Radiology. 2004;233(1):19.
4. Grimbizis GF, Camus M, Tarlatzis BC, Bontis JN, Delvoy P. Clinical implications of uterine malformations and hysteroscopic treatment results. Hum Reprod Update. 2001;7:161–74.
5. Rackow BW. Congenital uterine anomalies. In: Stadtmauer L, Tur-Kaspa I, editors. Ultrasound imaging in reproductive medicine: advances in infertility work-up, treatment and art. New York: Springer; 2014. p. 101–16.
6. Wu MH, Hsu CC, Huang KE. Detection of congenital müllerian duct anomalies using three-dimensional ultrasound. J Clin Ultrasound. 1997;25:487–92.
7. Reichman DE, Laufer MR. Congenital uterine anomalies affecting reproduction. Best Pract Res Clin Obstet Gynaecol. 2010;24:193–208.
8. Toaff ME, Lev-Toaff AS, Toaff R. Communicating uteri: review and classification with introduction of two previously unreported types. Fertil Steril. 1984;41:661–79.
9. Oppelt P, von Have M, Paulsen M, Strissel PL, Strick R, Brucker S, et al. Female genital malformations and their associated abnormalities. Fertil Steril. 2007;87:335–42.
10. Rackow BW, Arici A. Reproductive performance of women with müllerian anomalies. Curr Opin Obstet Gynecol. 2007;19(3):229–37.
11. Goldberg J, Falcone T. Mullerian anomalies: reproduction, diagnosis and treatment. In: Gidwani G,

Falcone T, editors. Congenital malformations of the female genital tract: diagnosis and management. Philadelphia: Lippincott Williams and Wilkins; 1999. p. 177–204.

12. Szkodziak P, Woźniak S, Czuczwar P, Paszkowski T, Milart P, Wozniakowska E, Szlichtyng W. Usefulness of three dimensional transvaginal ultrasonography and hysterosalpingography in diagnosing uterine anomalies. Ginekol Pol. 2014;85(5):354–9.

13. Salim R, Jurkovic D. Assessing congenital uterine anomalies: the role of three-dimensional ultrasonography. Best Pract Res Clin Obstet Gynecol. 2004; 18:29–36.

14. Moini A, Mohammadi S, Hosseini R, Eslami B, Ahmadi F. Accuracy of 3-dimensional sonography for diagnosis and classification of congenital uterine anomalies. J Ultrasound Med. 2013;32(6):923–7.

15. Ghi T, Casadio P, Kuleva M, Perrone AM, Savelli L, Giunchi S, et al. Accuracy of three-dimensional ultrasound in diagnosis and classification of congenital uterine anomalies. Fertil Steril. 2009;92:808–13.

16. Ludwin A, Pityński K, Ludwin I, Banas T, Knafel A. Two- and three-dimensional ultrasonography and sonohysterography versus hysteroscopy with laparoscopy in the differential diagnosis of septate, bicornuate, and arcuate uteri. J Minim Invasive Gynecol. 2013;20(1):90–9.

17. Faivre E, Fernandez H, Deffieux X, Gervaise A, Frydman R, Levaillant JM. Accuracy of three-dimensional ultrasonography in differential diagnosis of septate and bicornuate uterus compared with office hysteroscopy and pelvic magnetic resonance imaging. J Minim Invasive Gynecol. 2012;19(1):101–6.

18. Yoo RE, Cho JY, Kim SY, Kim SH. A systematic approach to the magnetic resonance imaging-based differential diagnosis of congenital Müllerian duct anomalies and their mimics. Abdom Imaging. 2015;40(1):192–206.

19. Bermejo C, Ten Martinez P, Cantarero R, Diaz D, Perez Pedregosa J, Barron E, et al. Three-dimensional ultrasound in the diagnosis of Müllerian duct anomalies and concordance with magnetic resonance imaging. Ultrasound Obstet Gynecol. 2010;35:593–601.

20. Lin PC, Bhatnagar KP, Nettleton GS, Nakajima ST. Female genital anomalies affecting reproduction. Fertil Steril. 2002;78:899–915.

21. Letterie G. Surgery, assisted reproductive technology and infertility: diagnosis and management of problems in gynecologic reproductive medicine. 2nd ed. Boca Raton: CRC; 2007. p. 149–80.

22. Rock JA, Breech LL. Surgery for anomalies of the mullerian ducts. In: Rock JA, Jones III HW, editors. Te Linde's operative gynaecology. 10th ed. Philadelphia: Lippincott-Williams & Wilkins; 2008. p. 572–5.

23. Lolis DE, Paschopoulos M, Makrydimas G, Zikopoulos K, Sotiriadis A, Paraskevaidis E. Reproductive outcome after Strassman metroplasty in women with a bicornuate uterus. J Reprod Med. 2005;50(5):297–301.

24. Rechberger T, Monist M, Bartuzi A. Clinical effectiveness of Strassman operation in the treatment of bicornuate uterus. Ginekol Pol. 2009;80(2):88–92.

25. Propst AM, Hill III JA. Anatomic factors associated with recurrent pregnancy loss. Semin Reprod Med. 2000;18:341–50.

26. Alborzi S, Asefjah H, Amini M, Vafaei H, Madadi G, Chubak N, Tavana Z. Laparoscopic metroplasty in bicornuate and didelphic uteri: feasibility and outcome. Arch Gynecol Obstet. 2015;291(5):1167–71.

27. Chan YY, Jayaprakasan K, Zamora J, Thornton JG, Raine-Fenning N, Coomarasamy A. The prevalence of congenital uterine anomalies in unselected and high-risk populations: a systematic review. Hum Reprod Update. 2011;17:761–71.

28. Hua M, Odibo A, Longman R, Macones G, Roehl K, Cahill A. Congential uterine anomalies and adverse pregnancy outcomes. Am J Obstet Gynecol. 2011;6:558.

29. Acien P. Reproductive performance of women with uterine malformations. Hum Reprod. 1993;8:122–6.

30. Heinonen PK, Saarikoski S, Pystynen P. Reproductive performance of women with uterine anomalies: an evaluation of 182 cases. Acta Obstet Gynecol Scand. 1982;61:157.

31. Raga F, Bauset C, Remohi J, Bonilla-Musoles F, Simon C, Pellicer A. Reproductive impact of congenital müllerian anomalies. Hum Reprod. 1997;12: 2277–81.

32. Yassaee F, Mostafaee L. The role of cervical cerclage in pregnancy outcome in women with uterine anomaly. J Reprod Infertil. 2011;12(4):277–9.

Uterus Didelphys: Diagnosis, Treatment, and Impact on Fertility and Reproduction

9

Joseph S. Sanfilippo and Kathryn Peticca

Incidence

Uterus didelphys results from the failed fusion of the paired Müllerian ducts. This creates two uterine horns with separate noncommunicating uterine cavities, each associated with its own uterine cervix and fallopian tube (Fig. 9.1). Uterus didelphys accounts for around 8–10 % of all Müllerian anomalies and occurs in approximately 1 in 3000 women [1, 2]. A longitudinal vaginal septum is found in up to 75 % of cases of uterus didelphys [3]. It is less common for a single vaginal canal to be present due to the embryologic origin of this condition.

As with all Müllerian anomalies, there is an association with renal anomalies. Unilateral renal anomalies can be found in 15–25 % of patients with uterus didelphys. These most frequently occur on the right side [4]. Renal agenesis is more commonly associated with uterus didelphys than with any other anomaly [5]. A rare condition called obstructed hemivagina and ipsilateral renal agenesis (OHVIRA), also known as Herlyn-Werner-Wunderlich (HWW) syndrome, is characterized by a triad of uterus didelphys, obstructed hemivagina, and ipsilateral renal agenesis [6]. This condition has been reported in 18 % of patients with uterus didelphys and is discussed in depth in Chap. 12 [7].

Differential Diagnosis

Uterus didelphys should be distinguished from complete septate uterus as well as bicornuate uterus or partial septate uterus. Uterus didelphys is often confused with a complete septate uterus because both have two cervices or cervical os and usually accompanied by a longitudinal vaginal septum. The difference is the shape of the upper uterus. Uterus didelphys describes a uterus with two separate often divergent uterine horns while complete septate uterus has a single uterine fundus with two separate endometrial cavities (Fig. 9.2). A bicornuate uterus and uterus didelphys have similar upper uterine shapes, but the difference lies with the cervix that is single with bicornuate and duplicated with didelphys. These can be distinguished by physical exam and imaging techniques such as US, 3D US, MRI, and HSG.

J.S. Sanfilippo, MD, MBA (✉) • K. Peticca, MD
University of Pittsburgh School of Medicine,
Magee-Womens Hospital, 300 Halket Street,
Pittsburgh, PA 15213, USA
e-mail: jsanfilippo@upmc.edu

© Springer International Publishing Switzerland 2016
S.M. Pfeifer (ed.), *Congenital Müllerian Anomalies*, DOI 10.1007/978-3-319-27231-3_9

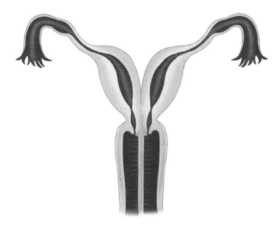

Fig. 9.1 Diagram of uterus didelphys with two separate uterine horns, two cervices and a longitudinal vaginal septum creating two vaginal cavities

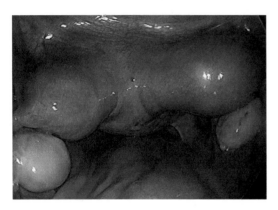

Fig. 9.2 Laparoscopic view of the outer uterine contour of a uterus didelphys. Note the uterine horns are separate and each has an adjacent ovary (*Image provided by Samantha M. Pfeifer MD*)

Diagnosis

Most patients with uterus didelphys are asymptomatic and go undiagnosed throughout their life, or are discovered incidentally during a fertility evaluation. Patients may present with obstetrical complications such as spontaneous abortions or preterm labor [2, 7]. Patients with an associated longitudinal vaginal septum more commonly present with symptoms such as vaginal discharge, dyspareunia as a result of a vaginal septum, or after the onset of menarche, with the inability of a tampon to obstruct menstrual flow due to two separate vaginal canals often described as "tampons don't work" [2].

When uterus didelphys is associated with a longitudinal vaginal septum, in rare instances, one of the hemivaginas can become obstructed by an oblique or transverse vaginal septum as is seen with OHVIRA/HWW syndromes [8]. In these instances, patients will become symptomatic after the onset of menarche presenting with increasingly severe dysmenorrhea or cyclic or continuous abdominal pain due to hematocolpos and hematometra [8]. However, diagnosis is often delayed months to years after menarche, as this condition is not considered in the differential diagnosis. Physical findings include unilateral lower abdominal tenderness, a palpable lower abdominal mass, or a vaginal mass on vaginal or rectal exam. Additionally, obstruction may result in endometriosis secondary to retrograde menstruation and is usually worse the longer the time between menarche and diagnosis [5] (Fig. 9.3).

A pelvic examination is important in the diagnosis of uterus didelphys. Careful vaginal examination should reveal the presence of two distinct cervices that can help differentiate uterus didelphys from bicornuate uterus. In addition, a longitudinal vaginal septum is present in the majority of cases. The septum may extend from the cervix down to the upper, mid, or lower vagina. In some cases, the septum may extend to the hymenal ring and the vaginal opening may be significantly smaller so that it may be difficult to see and therefore missed on exam.

If there is a duplicated cervix and longitudinal vaginal septum, then uterus didelphys must be distinguished from complete septate uterus. Initial screening with 2D ultrasound may differentiate septate from didelphys, as the uterine horns are usually disparate with didelphic uterus. If there is a single cervix on exam, then uterus didelphys is unlikely unless the vaginal septum and second vaginal canal was missed. For years, Magnetic Resonance Imaging (MRI) has been the gold standard imaging tool for diagnosing Müllerian anomalies with reported 100 % accuracy in differentiating between subtypes [9–11] (Fig. 9.4). It provides detailed information on the external and internal uterine contours, specifically of the uterine fundus, with excellent definition of the cervix and vagina [12]. However, recently, three-dimensional ultrasonography has begun to move to the

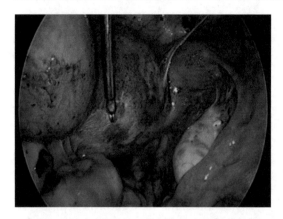

Fig. 9.3 Uterus didelphys with obstructed left hemivagina with distention of left vagina and left uterus with evidence of endometriosis due to retrograde menstruation from the obstruction. Note the normal size right uterine horn (*arrow*)

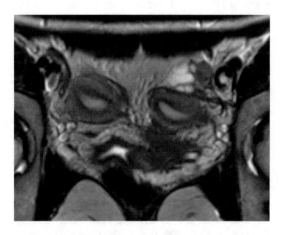

Fig. 9.4 MRI of uterus didelphys, Axial view demonstrating two disparate uterine horns (*Image provided by Samantha M. Pfeifer MD*)

forefront of diagnostic imaging with additional benefits of being less expensive, providing for more immediate results, and having a greater availability in the office. Although not as extensively studied as MRI, smaller studies have shown that it is comparable to MRI with reported accuracy of diagnosis between uterine subtypes ranging from 88 to 100 % [9, 10, 13–16]. Both of these techniques require interpretation by an experienced radiologist. With the advent of three-dimensional imaging, there is less of a need for

the use of exam under anesthesia and laparoscopy in diagnosis and should be reserved for more complex cases in which diagnosis is unclear (see Fig. 9.3). In cases of OHVIRA/HWW syndrome, MRI imaging is preferred due to the superior ability of MRI to evaluate and better characterize the vaginal canal and septum [12]. HSG may be helpful in determining the contour of the endometrial cavities and demonstrating tubal patency, but not in the adolescent. However, with a uterus didelphys both cervices need to be cannulated and would not necessarily differentiate complete septate uterus from uterus didelphys, as it does not capture the outer contour of the uterus.

All patients diagnosed with uterus didelphys should also undergo screening for renal anomalies with ultrasound. Additionally, any patient found to have a longitudinal vaginal septum should be evaluated for uterus didelphys and complete septate uterus due to the above mentioned high association between these conditions.

Treatment

Patients with uterus didelphys should be counseled that reproductive outcomes are overall favorable and surgical treatment to correct this anomaly is not advised. Pregnancy can occur in either of the two endometrial cavities. One study reported a greater incidence of pregnancy in the right uterine horn [7]. Due to the increased risk of preterm labor and malpresentation requiring a cesarean section, these patients should be considered high risk and followed closely. However, management of pregnancy in women with uterus didelphys is controversial with conflicting evidence. While many authors argue for interventions such as cerclages, use of 17-alpha hydroxyprogesterone, and scheduling a cesarean section versus trial of vaginal delivery, there is no evidence in the literature to support any of these measures for women with uterus didelphys.

There is no evidence to support the surgical treatment of uterus didelphys to improve pregnancy outcomes or fertility [5]. Although the Strassman metroplasty, typically utilized for

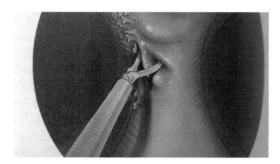

Fig. 9.5 Resecting the longitudinal vaginal septum. Typically the cut edges of the septum need to be cauterized or sutured for hemostasis

bicornuate uteri, has been used in the past to unify the didelphic cavities [17–19]. With the advances in obstetrical medicine, this procedure is rarely, if ever, indicated for uterus didelphys.

Patients who have an associated longitudinal vaginal septum may benefit from septum resection if symptomatic. Typical indication for surgical resection of a vaginal septum include the inability to use tampons, which may be a significant issue for many adolescents, dyspareunia, or a feeling of being "abnormal." Surgical correction is not mandatory. Resection of the vaginal septum can be accomplished by excising the septum along the anterior and posterior vaginal walls then marsupializing the edges of the two vaginal cavities along the anterior and posterior vagina with running locking or interrupted suture for hemostasis (Fig. 9.5). Alternatively, cautery or ligasure can be used. Simple incision of the septum is also an option but in some cases may result in excessive remnant vaginal tissue. Postoperative adhesions between anterior and posterior vaginal incision lines are rare.

Impact on Fertility and Reproduction

Müllerian anomalies in general have not been shown to be a cause of primary infertility although there are varying reports in the literature. In a study by Heinonen et al. following 49 women with uterus didelphys for a period of 9 years, they reported no impairment in primary infertility

within their small sample size [7]. There have been many additional small retrospective studies with differing reports although definitive conclusions cannot be drawn from these due to the small, retrospective nature of these studies. In a large retrospective analysis by Chan et al. following the outcomes of 3800 women with Müllerian anomalies, they found no statistically significant difference in the pregnancy rates of women with uterus didelphys versus that of women with normal uteri [20].

Uterus didelphys does affect obstetrical outcomes with typically a higher risk of preterm delivery and malpresentation compared to those with a normal uterus. However, as the literature is primarily small observational, retrospective studies the reported outcomes vary and conclusions difficult. A recent meta-analysis of published literature showed while uterus didelphys had a higher rate of preterm delivery <37 weeks gestation compared to other uterine anomalies, the rate of preterm delivery <28 weeks gestation and perinatal mortality was lower for uterus didelphys than for septate, bicornuate, unicornuate, or combined/undefined anomalies [21]. The improved reproductive outcome for uterus didelphys compared to unicornuate uterus has been hypothesized to be due to a better collateral blood supply between both uterine horns with uterus didelphys [22]. Multiple small retrospective studies evaluating reproductive outcomes of pregnant women with uterus didelphys have reported spontaneous abortion rates ranging from 20 to 43 % with one small study reporting 70 %, preterm delivery rates ranging from 21 to 53 %, term delivery rates ranging between 20 and 36 %, and live birth rates ranging from 40 to 75 % [1, 2, 5, 10, 18, 19, 23]. A high rate of a cesarean section has been noted in women with uterus didelphys. In one study of 33 women some of whom had more than one delivery, the cesarean rate was 84 % with 51 % of babies in the breech presentation [7]. In a systematic review by Chan et al, evaluating the reproductive outcomes of nine studies comprising over 3800 women they also found an increase in rate of preterm labor and fetal malpresentation in women with uterus didelphys [20].

References

1. Grimbizis GF, Camus M, Tarlatzis BC, Bontis JN, Devroey P. Clinical implications of uterine malformations and hysteroscopic treatment results. Hum Reprod Update. 2001;7(2):161–74.
2. Heinonen PK, Saarikoski S, Pystynen P. Reproductive performance of women with uterine anomalies. An evaluation of 182 cases. Acta Obstet Gynecol Scand. 1982;61(2):157–62.
3. Buttram VC. Müllerian anomalies and their management. Fertil Steril. 1983;40(2):159–63.
4. Vercellini P, Daguati R, Somigliana E, Viganò P, Lanzani A, Fedele L. Asymmetric lateral distribution of obstructed hemivagina and renal agenesis in women with uterus didelphys: institutional case series and a systematic literature review. Fertil Steril. 2007;87(4):719–24.
5. Lin PC. Reproductive outcomes in women with uterine anomalies. J Womens Health. 2004;13(1):33–9.
6. Humphries PD, Simpson JC, Creighton SM, Hall-Craggs MA. MRI in the assessment of congenital vaginal anomalies. Clin Radiol. 2008;63(4):442–8.
7. Heinonen PK. Clinical implications of the didelphic uterus: long-term follow-up of 49 cases. Eur J Obstet Gynecol Reprod Biol. 2000;91(2):183–90.
8. Stassart JP, Nagel TC, Prem KA, Phipps WR. Uterus didelphys, obstructed hemivagina, and ipsilateral renal agenesis: the University of Minnesota experience. Fertil Steril. 1992;57(4):756–61.
9. Pellerito JS, McCarthy SM, Doyle MB, Glickman MG, DeCherney AH. Diagnosis of uterine anomalies: relative accuracy of MR imaging, endovaginal sonography, and hysterosalpingography. Radiology. 1992;183(3):795–800.
10. Raga F, Bonilla-Musoles F, Blanes J, Osborne NG. Congenital Müllerian anomalies: diagnostic accuracy of three-dimensional ultrasound. Fertil Steril. 1996;65(3):523–8.
11. Deutch TD, Abuhamad AZ. The role of 3-dimensional ultrasonography and magnetic resonance imaging in the diagnosis of Müllerian duct anomalies: a review of the literature. J Ultrasound Med. 2008;27(3):412–23.
12. Bermejo C, Ten Martínez P, Cantarero R, Diaz D, Pérez Pedregosa J, Barrón E, Labrador E, Ruiz López L. Three-dimensional ultrasound in the diagnosis of Müllerian duct anomalies and concordance with magnetic resonance imaging. Ultrasound Obstet Gynecol. 2010;35:593–601.
13. Ghi T, Casdio P, Kuleva M, et al. Accuracy of three-dimensional ultrasound in diagnosis and classification of congenital uterine anomalies. Fertil Steril. 2009;92:808–13.
14. Bocca S, Oehinger S, Stadtmauer L, et al. A study of the cost, accuracy, and benefits of 3-dimensional sonography compared with hsyterosalpinography in women with uterine abnormalities. J Ultrasound Med. 2012;31:81–5.
15. Moini A, Mohammadi S, Hosseini R, Eslami B, Ahmadi F. Accuracy of 3-dimensional sonography for diagnosis and classification of congenital uterine anomalies. J Ultrasound Med. 2013;32(6):923–7.
16. Wu MH, HSU CC, Huang KE. Detection of congenital Müllerian duct anomalies using three-dimensional ultrasound. J Clin Ultrasound. 1997;25:487–92.
17. Steinberg W. Strassmann's metroplasty in the management of bipartite uterus causing sterility or habitual abortion. Obstet Gynecol Surv. 1955;10:400–30.
18. Fedele L, Amberletti D, Alberton A, Vercellin P, Candiani G. Gestational aspects of uterus didelphys. J Reprod Med. 1988;33(4):353–5.
19. Heinonen P. Uterus Didelphys: a report of 26 cases. Eur J Obstet Gynecol Reprod Biol. 1984;16(5):345–50.
20. Chan YY, Jayaprakasan K, Tan A, Thornton JG, Coomarasamy A, Raine-Fenning NJ. Reproductive outcomes in women with congenital uterine anomalies: a systematic review. Ultrasound Obstet Gynecol. 2011;38:371–82.
21. Venetis CA, Papadopoulos SP, Campo R, Gordts S, Tarlatzis BC, Grimbizis GF. Clinical implications of congenital uterine anomalies: a meta-analysis of comparative studies. Reprod Biomed Online. 2014;29:665–83.
22. Hoffman B, Schorge J, Schaffer J, Halvorson L, Bradshaw K, Cunningham G. Anatomic disorders. 2nd ed. New York: McGraw-Hill; 2012.
23. Hua M, Odibo AO, Longman RE, Macones GA, Roehl KA, Cahill AG. Congenital uterine anomalies and adverse pregnancy outcomes. Am J Obstet Gynecol. 2011;205:558.e1–5.

Unicornuate Uterus

Erica B. Mahany and Yolanda R. Smith

Prevalence

It is estimated that Müllerian duct anomalies are present in 0.3–10 % of all women [1–21]. In women with recurrent miscarriages (both first and second trimester), this number may be as high as 25–30 %[1, 3, 5–8, 13, 15, 19, 20]. It is reported that 5–20 % of Müllerian duct anomalies are the unicornuate uterus subtype [1, 2, 4, 10, 16, 20, 22]. If the distribution of these anomalies is not skewed based on poor pregnancy outcome, then approximately 1–6 % of women with recurrent miscarriages have a unicornuate uterus. Most studies looking at reproductive performance consider Müllerian duct anomalies in general, and do not stratify based on the unicornuate uterus subtype. Akar et al. reported that 3 % (55/1784) of patients presenting with infertility, recurrent pregnancy loss, pain, or acute abdomen, had a unicornuate uterus [10].

Etiology

The unicornuate uterus results from the normal development of one of the paired Müllerian ducts and incomplete or absent development of the contralateral duct. Four subtypes are classified based on the degree of developmental arrest in the contralateral duct [15, 19, 23–25]. A simple unicornuate uterus is present if there is no rudimentary horn (Fig. 10.1). The ipsilateral fallopian tube develops normally on this side. This scenario accounts for 35 % of patients with a unicornuate uterus. If a rudimentary horn is present, it may communicate with the main uterine cavity (10 % of patients with a unicornuate uterus), or it may be separate from the main uterine cavity, also called "noncommunicating." A noncommunicating horn may be classified further: if endometrium is present, it is cavitary (22 % of patients with a unicornuate uterus); if endometrium is absent, it is noncavitary (33 % of patients with a unicornuate uterus) [16, 26]. Among the four subtypes, development of the fallopian tube varies. As the ovaries are not Müllerian structures, ovarian development is usually normal, although they may be malpositioned. The ovaries may be found superior or inferior to the common iliac vessels, and they may be elongated [15, 16, 27, 28]. Anomalies of the urinary tract are also common. Renal agenesis contralateral to the main

E.B. Mahany, M.D. (✉) • Y.R. Smith, M.D., M.S.
L4510 Women's Hospital, 1500 East Medical
Center Drive, Ann Arbor, MI 48109, USA
e-mail: emahany@med.umich.edu;
ysmith@med.umich.edu

© Springer International Publishing Switzerland 2016
S.M. Pfeifer (ed.), *Congenital Müllerian Anomalies*, DOI 10.1007/978-3-319-27231-3_10

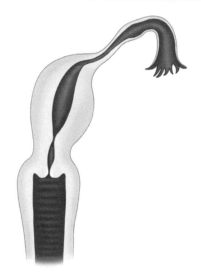

Fig. 10.1 Left unicornuate uterus

uterine horn is the most common abnormality, reported to be present in 28–67 % of patients with a unicornuate uterus [1, 10, 15, 19, 25, 26, 29–31].

The particular cause of the unicornuate uterus is unknown. Although increased occurrence risks for first-degree relatives suggest a role for genetic factors, a particular gene responsible for these malformations has not been found [2, 32]. One study evaluated 24 index cases and found 2.7 % (1/37) of sisters had a clinically significant uterine anomaly, suggesting a polygenic or multifactorial etiology [4, 15, 33]. Similarly, no associated environmental exposure has been found. Although it is clear that diethylstilbestrol and several other xenoestrogens disrupt the development of the female reproductive tract by altering HOX gene expression, there has been no particular compound found to cause unicornuate uterus in particular [34].

Differential Diagnosis

The clinical presentation of the unicornuate uterus depends on the particular subtype present. A simple unicornuate uterus is usually

asymptomatic and often comes to the attention of the provider only during evaluation for recurrent pregnancy loss, on imaging for another indication, during pregnancy, or at the time of cesarean delivery. The physical exam may be unreliable given that the deviation of the uterus to one side may be subtle. These patients will typically have a single vagina and a single cervix. Patients with rudimentary horn containing functional endometrium may present at menarche or later in life with dysmenorrhea primarily localized to the side of the rudimentary horn with associated hematometra or hematosalpinx. These individuals may also present with increasingly severe dysmenorrhea or chronic pelvic pain caused by retrograde menstruation and resulting endometriosis. Another group of patients may present with pregnancy-related complications such as first or second trimester abortions, preterm delivery, intrauterine fetal demise, or ectopic pregnancy in the fallopian tube contralateral to the unicornuate uterus [1, 15]. In addition, pregnancy can develop in the rudimentary horn, whether it is communicating to the main uterine cavity or not, the latter of which happens through transperitoneal migration of sperm. These pregnancies often rupture the uterine horn in which they are located, usually in the second trimester when the blood supply to the pregnancy is robust, which can lead to hemorrhagic shock and even death [1, 3, 30, 35].

If a unicornuate uterus is suspected on imaging, it must be differentiated from other Müllerian anomalies such as bicornuate uterus, septate uterus, and uterus didelphys [1]. These may be difficult to distinguish on modalities such as two-dimensional ultrasound or hysterosalpingogram (HSG). Magnetic resonance imaging (MRI) has traditionally been most useful in terms of an accurate diagnosis, although three-dimensional ultrasound is emerging as a similarly useful modality for this purpose [18, 36–42]. A noncommunicating, noncavity horn may be misdiagnosed as a fibroid or adnexal mass [42], and it is important to diagnose the rudimentary horn if present in order to prevent complications due to pelvic pain or an ectopic pregnancy.

Diagnosis

The workup for a Müllerian duct anomaly often begins with two-dimensional ultrasound or HSG; however, MRI or three-dimensional ultrasound is often needed to classify the Müllerian duct anomaly as these modalities allow for multiplanar imaging and evaluation of the fundal contour [19, 23, 26, 43].

The classic appearance of a unicornuate uterus on HSG includes a midline "banana-shaped" uterine cavity with contrast opacification of a solitary fallopian tube (Fig. 10.2). It may identify a communicating rudimentary horn if present [19]. On two-dimensional ultrasound, it appears as a small, oblong, off-midline structure. A rudimentary horn may be hard to identify [19, 26, 43]. On MRI, a unicornuate uterus appears as a small, curved hemi-uterus displaced off-midline. Myometrial zonal anatomy is normal [19, 36, 37] (Fig. 10.3). The rudimentary horn varies by subtype. If endometrial tissue is absent in the rudimentary horn, then zonal anatomy is absent and the entire horn may demonstrate low signal

intensity. If endometrial tissue is present, zonal anatomy may be preserved. The rudimentary horn may be distended with blood products in the case of an obstruction [19]. An additional benefit of MRI is that an evaluation may be performed simultaneously for renal anomalies as

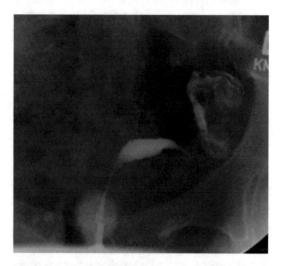

Fig. 10.2 HSG of Left unicornuate uterus (*image provided by Samantha M. Pfeifer M.D.*)

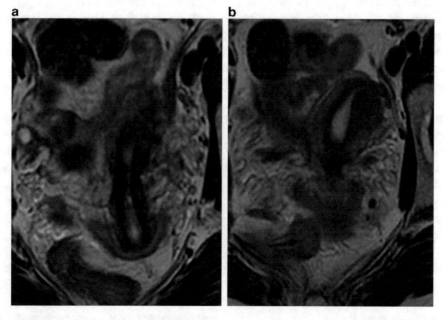

Fig. 10.3 MRI of Left unicornuate uterus. (**a**) Lower uterine segment and cervix. (**b**) Upper uterus. Note the cornual area (*Image provided by Samantha M.Pfeifer MD*)

ipsilateral renal agenesis is frequently present. Three-dimensional ultrasonography has similar sensitivity and specificity to MRI (approaching 100 %, respectively) [18, 38, 42, 43] and also has a similar ability to evaluate for a rudimentary horn. Sometimes, a unicornuate uterus is discovered at the time of office hysteroscopy during a workup for infertility or another indication such as abnormal uterine bleeding. Laparoscopy may also be useful to confirm the diagnosis, although with the high quality of multiplanar imaging modalities, this is usually unnecessary.

Therapy

A simple unicornuate uterus often needs no specific intervention other than counseling and referral to a high risk obstetrician, who may discuss further management in pregnancy. If a non-communicating rudimentary horn without endometrium is present, it may be left in place. A rudimentary horn with functional endometrium should be removed for three reasons: to minimize rupture of a rudimentary horn pregnancy, to promote conception in the unicornuate cavity, and to minimize dysmenorrhea symptoms as well as endometriosis and adhesive disease associated with increased cavity distention and retrograde menstruation [2, 3, 5, 15, 19, 29, 35, 44, 45]. If a rudimentary horn is removed, the ipsilateral fallopian tube should also be removed to prevent an ectopic pregnancy in that fallopian tube [45]. What is not clear, however, is whether to remove the fallopian tube contralateral to an asymptomatic unicornuate uterus. Although an ectopic pregnancy may occur in this fallopian tube, the existing data do not suggest an increased ectopic pregnancy rate in these situations [29]. Patients should be counseled regarding the possibility of an ectopic occurring in the contralateral fallopian tube as this diagnosis may be overlooked. However, in a patient with a BRCA mutation, salpingectomy may be performed as part of a strategy to reduce the risk of future ovarian and fallopian tube cancer [46].

Impact on Fertility/Reproduction

It is well documented that women with unicornuate uteri have increased pregnancy complications, such as first trimester miscarriages, second trimester miscarriages, preterm delivery, intrauterine growth restriction, and malpresentation [1, 2, 4, 5, 7, 10, 12, 20, 29, 45, 47–49]. Chan performed a systematic review evaluating 3805 subjects with a congenital uterine anomaly. The relative risk in patients with a unicornuate uterus for first trimester miscarriage compared to controls was 2.15, for second trimester miscarriage was 2.22, for preterm birth was 3.47, and for malpresentation was 2.74. Live birth rates have ranged from 30 to 66 %[5, 7, 10, 29, 49, 50]. The proposed mechanisms for these sequelae include abnormal uterine vasculature, cervical incompetence, and decreased muscle mass of the unicornuate uterus leading to second trimester abortion and preterm delivery [5, 15].

Cerclage has been attempted in women with a unicornuate uterus. Two studies have shown promising results in patients with uterine anomalies, although both were underpowered to draw conclusions about a unicornuate uterus in particular, and neither was randomized [15]. In 1983, Ambramovici et al. evaluated 15 patients with subfertility as a result of a congenital uterine anomaly who had cerclage placed at 11–12 weeks of gestation. The spontaneous abortion rate decreased from 88 to 0 %, and the term delivery rate increased from 0 to 87 % after placement of cerclage. Of the two women who delivered prematurely, their babies were alive and well at the time the study was published. They concluded that cerclage should be placed in cases of diminished fertility as a result of a congenital uterine anomaly [51]. In 1990, Golan et al. evaluated 29 cases of cervical incompetence in 98 women with a congenital uterine anomaly. They found an improvement in obstetrical performance following cerclage. In the cervical incompetence group, term deliveries increased from 26 to 63 %. Even in women with an anomalous uterus without proven diagnosis of cervical incompetence, term deliveries increased from 64 to 96 % [52]. They concluded that cerclage should be placed in women with a bicornuate uterus (as outcomes were worst in this subgroup) and that cerclage in all cases of uterine anomalies should be considered.

In addition, there are some data to suggest that women with a unicornuate uterus have a more difficult time achieving conception [15, 20]. In Chan's systematic review, the relative risk for conception was 0.74 compared with controls [13]. Some women with a unicornuate uterus may need assistance to achieve a pregnancy. As most fertility treatments utilize medications that increase the risk of multiple gestation, care should be taken in a woman with a unicornuate uterus as multifetal gestation would increase the risks of preterm delivery and pregnancy complications. For those women undergoing in vitro fertilization (IVF), it is important to consider elective single embryo transfer.

Several studies have evaluated the differences between women with and without a congenital uterine anomaly undergoing assisted reproductive technology (ART). While some show no impact on pregnancy rates, the studies are all observational, making conclusions difficult. Marcus et al. (1996) evaluated 24 patients with a congenital uterine anomaly who underwent IVF at a tertiary care center. Only 6 of these patients had a unicornuate uterus. The clinical pregnancy rate was 19 of 51 (37.9 %) per embryo transfer and 17 of 24 (70.8 %) per patient. There were no significant differences in the clinical pregnancy rates between different Müllerian anomalies, and the mean number of embryos transferred ranged from 2.7 to 2.9 [53]. Jayaprakasan et al. (2011) prospectively evaluated 1402 subjects undergoing ART and performed three-dimensional ultrasound to diagnose uterine anomalies, which were demonstrated in 184 (13.3 %) subjects. There were only 6 patients with unicornuate uterus. They found that patients with uterine anomalies had similar pregnancy rates to matched controls with normal uteri, although women with major uterine anomalies had a higher miscarriage rate (42.9 %) [14].

Heinonen et al. looked at IVF pregnancy outcomes compared to a historical control group [20]. This study only evaluated 17 patients undergoing 55 IVF cycles, 8 of whom had a unicornuate uterus. In the population of women with a unicornuate uterus specifically, pregnancy rate per embryo transfer was 19.4 %, although no control data were provided [20]. They also found an unusually high ectopic pregnancy rate of 33 % (2/6 patients). Patients with a unicornuate uterus had a lower delivery rate per embryo transfer (5.0 %) compared with a historical database at the same facility (17.5–19.0 %) [54].

Lavergne et al. evaluated 38 subjects undergoing 119 oocyte retrievals, and compared the pregnancy outcomes with a French national database during the same time period, from 1987 to 1992. Seventeen of these patients had a unicornuate uterus. Patients in the uterine anomaly group responded similarly well to controlled ovarian hyperstimulation. The number of transferred embryos was comparable between the study and control groups (2.85 vs. 2.86). These were most likely cleavage stage embryos, considering when the study was performed. They found that patients with a uterine anomaly had lower pregnancy rate per oocyte retrieval (11.7 % vs. 19.1 %, $p < 0.01$), lower pregnancy rate per embryo transfer (13.6 % vs. 24.9 %, $p < 0.01$), and lower implantation rate (5.8 % vs. 11.7 %, $p < 0.01$) [55].

As this anomaly is relatively uncommon, the small sample size makes it difficult to draw conclusions. A large multicenter study is necessary to capture enough women to address this concern with statistical significance.

It is important to counsel patients with a unicornuate uterus that the prognosis for them may still be good, even in the face of recurrent losses. Sugiura-Ogasawara et al. evaluated the pregnancy outcomes of 1676 patients with a history of two or more (2–12) consecutive miscarriages [56]. Fifty-four (3.2 %) of these women had congenital uterine anomalies, 5 of whom had a unicornuate uterus. Of the patients with a unicornuate uterus, one succeeded in having an infant with the first pregnancy after evaluation, and four of five had an infant cumulatively.

Although achieving a pregnancy may not be a problem for these women, these women are at risk for miscarriage, preterm delivery, and malpresentation. Data are lacking regarding methods to reduce preterm delivery such as the use of cerclage or progesterone. More studies must be done to elucidate the mechanism of poor pregnancy outcome in these patients in order to improve the treatments offered.

References

1. Khati NJ, Frazier AA, Brindle KA. The unicornuate uterus and its variants: clinical presentation, imaging findings, and associated complications. J Ultrasound Med. 2012;31(2):319–31.
2. Brucker SY, Rall K, Campo R, Oppelt P, Isaacson K. Treatment of congenital malformations. Semin Reprod Med. 2011;29(2):101–12. PubMed Epub 2011/03/26.eng.
3. Robbins JB, Parry JP, Guite KM, Hanson ME, Chow LC, Kliewer MA, et al. MRI of pregnancy-related issues: mullerian duct anomalies. AJR Am J Roentgenol. 2012;198(2):302–10. PubMed Epub 2012/01/24.eng.
4. Nahum GG. Uterine anomalies. How common are they, and what is their distribution among subtypes? J Reprod Med. 1998;43(10):877–87. PubMed Epub 1998/11/04.eng.
5. Rackow BW, Arici A. Reproductive performance of women with mullerian anomalies. Curr Opin Obstet Gynecol. 2007;19(3):229–37. PubMed Epub 2007/05/15.eng.
6. Acien P, Acien M. Unilateral renal agenesis and female genital tract pathologies. Acta Obstet Gynecol Scand. 2010;89(11):1424–31. PubMed Epub 2010/08/31.eng.
7. Grimbizis GF, Camus M, Tarlatzis BC, Bontis JN, Devroey P. Clinical implications of uterine malformations and hysteroscopic treatment results. Hum Reprod Update. 2001;7(2):161–74. PubMed Epub 2001/04/04.eng.
8. Raga F, Bauset C, Remohi J, Bonilla-Musoles F, Simon C, Pellicer A. Reproductive impact of congenital Mullerian anomalies. Hum Reprod. 1997;12(10):2277–81. PubMed Epub 1997/12/24.eng.
9. Simon C, Martinez L, Pardo F, Tortajada M, Pellicer A. Mullerian defects in women with normal reproductive outcome. Fertil Steril. 1991;56(6):1192–3. PubMed Epub 1991/12/01.eng.
10. Akar ME, Bayar D, Yildiz S, Ozel M, Yilmaz Z. Reproductive outcome of women with unicornuate uterus. Aust N Z J Obstet Gynaecol. 2005;45(2):148–50. PubMed Epub 2005/03/12.eng.
11. Forstner R, Hricak H. Congenital malformations of uterus and vagina. Radiologe. 1994;34(7):397–404. PubMed Epub 1994/07/01.eng.
12. Maneschi F, Zupi E, Marconi D, Valli E, Romanini C, Mancuso S. Hysteroscopically detected asymptomatic mullerian anomalies. Prevalence and reproductive implications. J Reprod Med. 1995;40(10):684–8. PubMed Epub 1995/10/01.eng.
13. Chan YY, Jayaprakasan K, Tan A, Thornton JG, Coomarasamy A, Raine-Fenning NJ. Reproductive outcomes in women with congenital uterine anomalies: a systematic review. Ultrasound Obstet Gynecol. 2011;38(4):371–82. PubMed Epub 2011/08/11.eng.
14. Jayaprakasan K, Chan YY, Sur S, Deb S, Clewes JS, Raine-Fenning NJ. Prevalence of uterine anomalies and their impact on early pregnancy in women conceiving after assisted reproduction treatment. Ultrasound Obstet Gynecol. 2011;37(6):727–32. PubMed Epub 2011/02/22.eng.
15. Reichman D, Laufer MR, Robinson BK. Pregnancy outcomes in unicornuate uteri: a review. Fertil Steril. 2009;91(5):1886–94. PubMed Epub 2008/04/29.eng.
16. Brody JM, Koelliker SL, Frishman GN. Unicornuate uterus: imaging appearance, associated anomalies, and clinical implications. AJR Am J Roentgenol. 1998;171(5):1341–7. PubMed Epub 1998/11/03. eng.
17. Zanetti E, Ferrari LR, Rossi G. Classification and radiographic features of uterine malformations: hysterosalpingographic study. Br J Radiol. 1978;51(603):161–70. PubMed Epub 1978/03/01. eng.
18. Deutch TD, Abuhamad AZ. The role of 3-dimensional ultrasonography and magnetic resonance imaging in the diagnosis of mullerian duct anomalies: a review of the literature. J Ultrasound Med. 2008;27(3):413–23. PubMed Epub 2008/03/04.eng.
19. Behr SC, Courtier JL, Qayyum A. Imaging of mullerian duct anomalies. Radiographics. 2012;32(6): E233–50. PubMed Epub 2012/10/16.eng.
20. Lin PC. Reproductive outcomes in women with uterine anomalies. J Womens Health. 2004;13(1):33–9. PubMed Epub 2004/03/10.eng.
21. Fritz MA, Speroff L. Clinical gynecologic endocrinology and infertility. 8th ed. Philadelphia: Lippincott Williams & Wilkins; 2011.
22. Medeiros LR, Rosa DD, Silva FR, Silva BR, Rosa MI. Laparoscopic approach of a unicornuate uterus with noncommunicating rudimentary horns. ISRN Obstet Gynecol. 2011;2011:906138. PubMed PMCID: Pmc3101792. Epub 2011/06/08.eng.
23. Yoo RE, Cho JY, Kim SY, Kim SH. A systematic approach to the magnetic resonance imaging-based differential diagnosis of congenital Mullerian duct anomalies and their mimics. Abdom Imaging. 2015; 40(1):192–206. PubMed Epub 2014/07/30.Eng.
24. Marten K, Vosshenrich R, Funke M, Obenauer S, Baum F, Grabbe E. MRI in the evaluation of mullerian duct anomalies. Clin Imaging. 2003;27(5):346–50. PubMed Epub 2003/08/23.eng.

25. Buttram Jr VC, Gibbons WE. Mullerian anomalies: a proposed classification. (An analysis of 144 cases). Fertil Steril. 1979;32(1):40–6. PubMed Epub 1979/07/01.eng.

26. Troiano RN, McCarthy SM. Mullerian duct anomalies: imaging and clinical issues. Radiology. 2004;233(1):19–34. PubMed Epub 2004/08/20.eng.

27. Ombelet W, Verswijvel G, Vanholsbeke C, Schobbens JC. Unicornuate uterus and ectopic (undescended) ovary. Facts Views Vis Obgyn. 2011;3(2):131–4. PubMed PMCID: Pmc3987487. Epub 2011/01/01.eng.

28. Allen JW, Cardall S, Kittijarukhajorn M, Siegel CL. Incidence of ovarian maldescent in women with mullerian duct anomalies: evaluation by MRI. AJR Am J Roentgenol. 2012;198(4):W381–5. PubMed Epub 2012/03/28.eng.

29. Heinonen PK. Unicornuate uterus and rudimentary horn. Fertil Steril. 1997;68(2):224–30. PubMed Epub 1997/08/01.eng.

30. Heinonen PK. Clinical implications of the unicornuate uterus with rudimentary horn. Int J Gynaecol Obstet. 1983;21(2):145–50. PubMed Epub 1983/04/01.eng.

31. Fedele L, Bianchi S, Agnoli B, Tozzi L, Vignali M. Urinary tract anomalies associated with unicornuate uterus. J Urol. 1996;155(3):847–8. PubMed Epub 1996/03/01.eng.

32. Simpson JL. Genetics of female infertility due to anomalies of the ovary and mullerian ducts. Methods Mol Biol. 2014;1154:39–73. PubMed Epub 2014/05/02.eng.

33. Elias S, Simpson JL, Carson SA, Malinak LR, Buttram Jr VC. Genetics studies in incomplete mullerian fusion. Obstet Gynecol. 1984;63(3):276–9. PubMed Epub 1984/03/01.eng.

34. Toppari J. Environmental endocrine disrupters and disorders of sexual differentiation. Semin Reprod Med. 2002;20(3):305–12. PubMed Epub 2002/11/13.eng.

35. Jayasinghe Y, Rane A, Stalewski H, Grover S. The presentation and early diagnosis of the rudimentary uterine horn. Obstet Gynecol. 2005;105(6):1456–67. PubMed Epub 2005/06/04.eng.

36. Carrington BM, Hricak H, Nuruddin RN, Secaf E, Laros Jr RK, Hill EC. Mullerian duct anomalies: MR imaging evaluation. Radiology. 1990;176(3):715–20. PubMed Epub 1990/09/01.eng.

37. Pellerito JS, McCarthy SM, Doyle MB, Glickman MG, DeCherney AH. Diagnosis of uterine anomalies: relative accuracy of MR imaging, endovaginal sonography, and hysterosalpingography. Radiology. 1992;183(3):795–800. PubMed Epub 1992/06/01.eng.

38. Salim R, Jurkovic D. Assessing congenital uterine anomalies: the role of three-dimensional ultrasonography. Best Pract Res Clin Obstet Gynaecol. 2004;18(1):29–36. PubMed Epub 2004/05/05.eng.

39. Salim R, Woelfer B, Backos M, Regan L, Jurkovic D. Reproducibility of three-dimensional ultrasound diagnosis of congenital uterine anomalies. Ultrasound Obstet Gynecol. 2003;21(6):578–82. PubMed Epub 2003/06/17.eng.

40. Kupesic S. Clinical implications of sonographic detection of uterine anomalies for reproductive outcome. Ultrasound Obstet Gynecol. 2001;18(4):387–400. PubMed Epub 2002/01/10.eng.

41. Wu MH, Hsu CC, Huang KE. Detection of congenital mullerian duct anomalies using three-dimensional ultrasound. J Clin Ultrasound. 1997;25(9):487–92. PubMed Epub 1997/11/14.eng.

42. Devine K, McCluskey T, Henne M, Armstrong A, Venkatesan AM, Decherney A. Is magnetic resonance imaging sufficient to diagnose rudimentary uterine horn? A case report and review of the literature. J Minim Invasive Gynecol. 2013;20(4):533–6. PubMed PMCID: Pmc3720688. Epub 2013/03/29.eng.

43. Bermejo C, Ten Martinez P, Cantarero R, Diaz D, Perez Pedregosa J, Barron E, et al. Three-dimensional ultrasound in the diagnosis of Mullerian duct anomalies and concordance with magnetic resonance imaging. Ultrasound Obstet Gynecol. 2010;35(5):593–601. PubMed Epub 2010/01/07.eng.

44. Liu MM. Unicornuate uterus with rudimentary horn. Int J Gynaecol Obstet. 1994;44(2):149–53. PubMed Epub 1994/02/01.eng.

45. Fedele L, Bianchi S, Zanconato G, Berlanda N, Bergamini V. Laparoscopic removal of the cavitated noncommunicating rudimentary uterine horn: surgical aspects in 10 cases. Fertil Steril. 2005;83(2):432–6. PubMed Epub 2005/02/12.eng.

46. Sherman ME, Piedmonte M, Mai PL, Ioffe OB, Ronnett BM, Van Le L, et al. Pathologic findings at risk-reducing salpingo-oophorectomy: primary results from Gynecologic Oncology Group Trial GOG-0199. J Clin Oncol. 2014;32(29):3275–83. PubMed PMCID: Pmc4178524. Epub 2014/09/10.eng.

47. Donderwinkel PF, Dorr JP, Willemsen WN. The unicornuate uterus: clinical implications. Eur J Obstet Gynecol Reprod Biol. 1992;47(2):135–9. PubMed Epub 1992/11/19.eng.

48. Moutos DM, Damewood MD, Schlaff WD, Rock JA. A comparison of the reproductive outcome between women with a unicornuate uterus and women with a didelphic uterus. Fertil Steril. 1992;58(1):88–93. PubMed Epub 1992/07/01.eng.

49. Fedele L, Zamberletti D, Vercellini P, Dorta M, Candiani GB. Reproductive performance of women with unicornuate uterus. Fertil Steril. 1987;47(3):416–9. PubMed Epub 1987/03/01.eng.

50. Heinonen PK, Saarikoski S, Pystynen P. Reproductive performance of women with uterine anomalies. An evaluation of 182 cases. Acta Obstet Gynecol Scand. 1982;61(2):157–62. PubMed Epub 1982/01/01.eng.

51. Abramovici H, Faktor JH, Pascal B. Congenital uterine malformations as indication for cervical suture (cerclage) in habitual abortion and premature delivery. Int J Fertil. 1983;28(3):161–4. PubMed Epub 1983/01/01.eng.

52. Golan A, Langer R, Wexler S, Segev E, Niv D, David MP. Cervical cerclage—its role in the pregnant anomalous uterus. Int J Fertil. 1990;35(3):164–70. PubMed Epub 1990/05/01.eng.

53. Marcus S, al-Shawaf T, Brinsden P. The obstetric outcome of in vitro fertilization and embryo transfer in women with congenital uterine malformation. Am J Obstet Gynecol. 1996;175(1):85–9. PubMed Epub 1996/07/01.eng.

54. Heinonen PK, Kuismanen K, Ashorn R. Assisted reproduction in women with uterine anomalies. Eur J Obstet Gynecol Reprod Biol. 2000;89(2):181–4. PubMed Epub 2000/03/22.eng.

55. Lavergne N, Aristizabal J, Zarka V, Erny R, Hedon B. Uterine anomalies and in vitro fertilization: what are the results? Eur J Obstet Gynecol Reprod Biol. 1996;68(1–2):29–34. PubMed Epub 1996/09/01. eng.

56. Sugiura-Ogasawara M, Ozaki Y, Katano K, Suzumori N, Mizutani E. Uterine anomaly and recurrent pregnancy loss. Semin Reprod Med. 2011;29(6):514–21. PubMed Epub 2011/12/14.eng.

Noncommunicating Rudimentary Uterine Horns

11

Kate McCracken and S. Paige Hertweck

Incidence

A unicornuate uterus, as shown in Fig. 11.1, occurs with a frequency that ranges from 1 in 1000 [1] to 1 in 5400 women [2] and 74–90 % of those women with a unicornuate uterus will have an associated rudimentary uterine horn that may or may not communicate with the unicornuate uterus [2, 3].

These rudimentary horns may or may not have functional endometrium. Literature reports that approximately 55 % of rudimentary horns are noncommunicating and have functional endometrium [2]. Although classically listed as a single entity of ASRM Type IIA1b (Table 11.1), these can have varied appearances (Fig. 11.2).

Likewise, the appearance of ASRM Type IIA communicating horns can vary (Fig. 11.3).

Furthermore, rudimentary horns may consist of solid muscle, areas of adenomyosis, or hypoplastic tissue [3] (Fig. 11.4).

As a result of this, multiple terms have been used to describe these anomalies: unicornuate uterus with rudimentary horn, uterus bicornis unicollis with rudimentary horn, uterus bicornis unicollis with atretic horn, bicornuate uterus with accessory horn, and uterus bicornis unilatere rudimentarius. Such terms are all used interchangeably in the medical literature [4].

Etiology

Mullerian anomalies result from incomplete development of the mullerian ducts during weeks 7–8 of gestation, and are further complicated by variable failure of developmental progression and fusion up to 14 weeks gestation [5, 6].

Unicornuate uteri with a rudimentary horn result from the normal development of one mullerian duct coupled with the failure of the contralateral duct to elongate or to reach the urogenital sinus which forms the lower third of the vagina. These events take place in the ninth week of gestation.

There is a right-sided predominance of noncommunicating rudimentary horns that may be due to the left Mullerian duct advancing slightly ahead of the right [7]. A unicornuate uterus may also be caused by complete agenesis of all the organs derived from one urogenital ridge, resulting in a unicornuate uterus and the absence of both ovarian and Mullerian tissue on the contralateral side [1, 3].

K. McCracken, M.D. (✉) • S.P. Hertweck, M.D. (✉)
Kosair Children's Hospital Gynecology Specialists,
Norton Medical Plaza 2 - St. Matthews, Suite 303,
3991 Dutchmans Lane, Louisville, KY 40207, USA
e-mail: k.a.mccracken@hotmail.com;
paige.hertweck@nortonhealthcare.org

© Springer International Publishing Switzerland 2016
S.M. Pfeifer (ed.), *Congenital Müllerian Anomalies*, DOI 10.1007/978-3-319-27231-3_11

Differential Diagnosis

The differential diagnosis of obstructed blind ending or noncommunicating rudimentary uterine horns includes other uterine anomalies/conditions such as bicornuate uteri with either a large cavity or adenomyosis, or a septate uterus with an obstructed horn. Recently, there have been case reports describing cavitated accessory uterine masses in women with an otherwise normal uterus, suggestive of a new type of Mullerian anomaly [8, 9]. These described lesions are distinguished from blind ending horns in that they are isolated accessory masses lined with normal endometrium that occur in the presence of a normal uterus with bilateral fallopian tubes and ovaries. These cavitary accessory lesions typically

occur at the anterior uterus, near the round ligament (Figs. 11.5 and 11.6).

Another lesion that could be confused with a noncommunicating rudimentary uterine horn

Table 11.1 American Society for Reproductive Medicine (ASRM) classification of Mullerian anomalies

Class	Type of Mullerian structure
I	Mullerian agenesis or hypoplasia
	(A) Vaginal
	(B) Cervical
	(C) Fundal
	(D) Tubal
	(E) Combined
II	Unicornuate uterus
	(A1) Rudimentary horn with endometrial tissue
	(a) Communicating with the main uterine cavity
	(b) Not communicating with the main uterine cavity
	(A2) Rudimentary horn without endometrial cavity
	(B) No rudimentary horn
III	Didelphic uterus
IV	Bicornuate uterus
	(A) Complete
	(B) Partial
V	Septate uterus
	(A) Complete
	(B) Partial
VI	Arcuate uterus
VII	Diethylstilbestrol (DES)-related anomalies
	(A) T-shaped uterus
	(B) T-shaped uterus with dilated uterine horns
	(C) Uterine hypoplasia

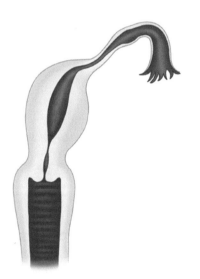

Fig. 11.1 Unicornuate uterus

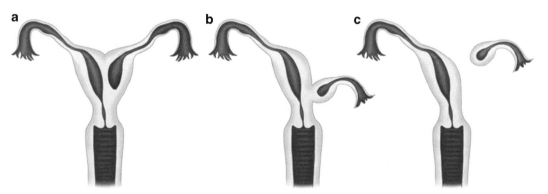

Fig. 11.2 Noncommunicating rudimentary horns with functional endometrium. Non-separated (**a**, **b**) and separated (**c**)

Fig. 11.3
Communicating
rudimentary horns.
Non-separated (**a**) and
separated (**b**)

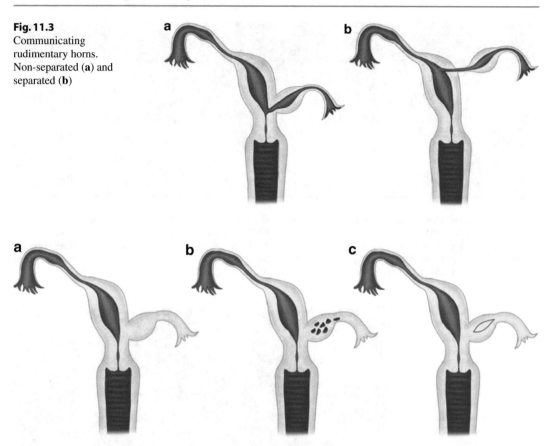

Fig. 11.4 Rudimentary uterine horns with endometrial anomaly: solid (**a**), adenomyosis (**b**), and hypoplasia (**c**)

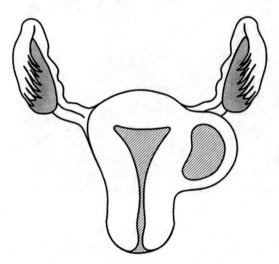

Fig. 11.5 Illustration of an anomaly with the anterior fundal bulge near the insertion of the left fallopian tube. (Potter DA, Schenken RS. Noncommunicating accessory uterine cavity. Fertil Steril 1998;70:1165-1166)

is the adenomyoma or cystic adenomyosis. Adenomyosis is characterized by invasion of the myometrium by endometrial tissue. These are frequently associated with leiomyomas. On histopathology, adenomyomas are notable for adenomyosis and an absence of internal epithelial lining. With imaging, it can be difficult to determine adenomyomas from an obstructed rudimentary horn (Fig. 11.7), but on laparoscopy or hysterosalpingogram, a normal uterus with bilateral fallopian tubes will be present in addition to the cavitary lesion [10] (Fig. 11.8).

Leiomyomata presentations can be confused with uterine horns, and imaging features can vary and make interpretation difficult. Necrotic and degenerating myomas can mimic hydrometra and pelvic malignancy [11], and the definitive diagnosis may only be made at the time of surgery.

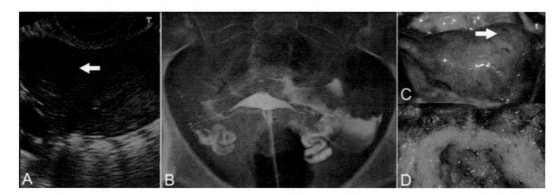

Fig. 11.6 (**a**) Transvaginal ultrasound image showing a cavitated uterine horn (*arrow*). (**b**) Hysterosalpingogram showing a normal uterus and tubes. (**c**) Photograph showing the leiomyoma-like nodule on the right anterior surface of the uterine fundus (*arrow*). (**d**) Surgical specimen after excision. A section of the tumor shows the internal endometrial lining of the tumor cavity. (Acien P, Acien M, Fernandez et al. The cavitated accessory uterine mass: a mullerian anomaly in women with an otherwise normal uterus. Obstet Gynecol 2010;116:1101-1109)

Fig. 11.7 Coronal MRI image demonstrating the cystic intramyometrial mass in the left anterior of the uterine body. (Dogen E, Gode F, Saatli B, Secil M. Juvenile cystic adenomyosis mimicking uterine malformation: a case report. Arch Gynecol Obstet 2008;278:593-595)

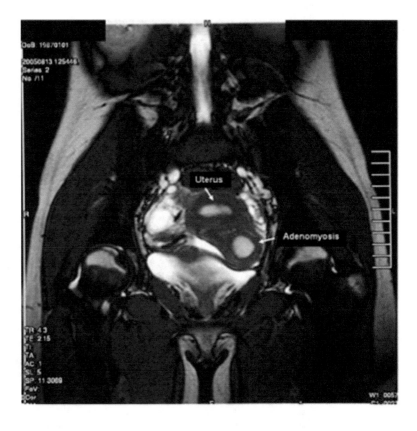

While noncommunicating rudimentary uterine horns are primarily classified under anomalies associated only with the unicornuate uterus (ASRM Type II), these anomalies may not fit into the traditional categories of classification. Rudimentary horns may be noted with uterovaginal agenesis (ASRM Type I) and may also occur in isolation without the presence of a unicornuate uterus (no existing ASRM classification). Additionally, bicornuate or septate uteri

Fig. 11.8 Laparoscopic appearance of the cystic adenomyosis. (Dogen E, Gode F, Saatli B, Secil M. Juvenile cystic adenomyosis mimicking uterine malformation: a case report. Arch Gynecol Obstet 2008;278:593-595)

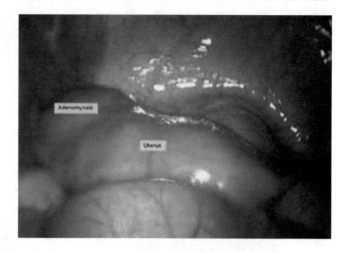

with hemi-obstruction are sometimes referred to as rudimentary horns and as type IV and V anomalies [3]. Important considerations for management of obstructed horns are the extent of endometrial activity within the horn and the degree of separation from other uterine structures that are present (see Fig. 2.4).

Obstructive Mullerian anomalies may vary somewhat in their presentations. While they have been reported in pre-menarchal girls [12], they typically present as pelvic pain, dysmenorrhea, or dyspareunia in the post-menarchal patient. The pain may be acute or chronic; and traditionally has been thought to be due to the absent outflow tract for functional endometrium. However, even non-cavitary, nonfunctional horns, in which pressure atrophy and adenomyosis has been excluded, can cause pain and patients have reported symptom resolution upon removal [13, 14].

A review of 366 cases of rudimentary uterine horns revealed that the mean age of presentation occurred in the early twenties, regardless of if the patient presented with a gynecologic or obstetric complaint (ages 23 and 26 years, respectively) [3]. This extensive review further noted that presentation in the third decade of life or later occurred in 78 % of patients. The time from onset of symptoms to presentation can vary and has been noted to be from 3 months to 18 years in one review [15].

Hospital presentations of women ultimately diagnosed with rudimentary horns have included

ectopic pregnancy (25 %), chronic pelvic pain (20 %), pelvic mass (20 %), and primary infertility (15 %) [16].

At the time of presentation, there may or may not be a pelvic mass present. The diagnosis may be delayed due to the presence of normal menstruation from the unobstructed uterus. Any patient with dysmenorrhea that fails to respond to typical medical management for primary dysmenorrhea should have an imaging study performed to evaluate for a rudimentary horn [17]. Noncommunicating rudimentary uterine horns have on rare occasion presented as inguinal masses or hernias with menstrual-related inguinal pain [18].

Diagnosis

MRI should be the imaging study of choice when one suspects a noncommunicating rudimentary uterine horn. MRI is a noninvasive method that will provide evaluation of both the internal and external morphology of the uterus. It has a high reported sensitivity 73–100 % in assessing women with surgically proven uterine anomalies [19, 20], and it has high resolution for soft tissues. The T2 weighted images are helpful for the diagnosis of uterine anomalies [21]; images on the sagittal and coronal sections can be used to evaluate the cervical anatomy. T1 weighted images are helpful in diagnosing endometriomas

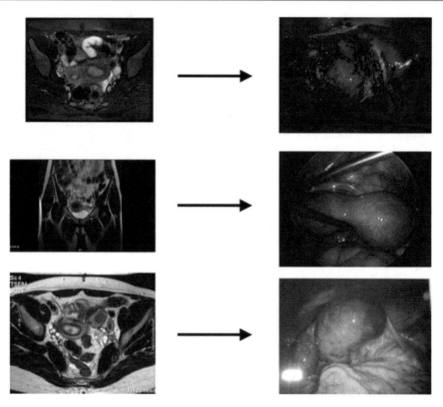

Fig. 11.9 Preoperative MRIs anticipating the surgical complexity in three cases and surgical images from the same cases showing the extent of myometrial connections. (Spitzer RF, Kives S, Allen L. Case series of laparoscopically resected noncommunicating functional uterine horns. J Pediatr Adoles Gynecol 2009;22:e23-e28)

[22] that may be associated findings in cases of obstructive Mullerian anomalies.

MRI is particularly helpful in identifying if functional endometrium is present within the rudimentary horn. Furthermore, it may allow the surgeon to anticipate the degree of myometrial connection between the noncommunicating horn and the unicornuate uterus—i.e., whether they are separate, joined by a thin filmy band, or fused [23]. The images in Fig. 11.9 illustrate this by contrasting the preoperative MRI and their correlated intraoperative images of three cases of noncommunicating functional uterine horns [23].

While MRI is a sensitive test, it is not perfect—many lateral defects may be missed [24–26], and the delineation between septate and bicornuate uteri may be challenging and dependent upon the expertise of the radiologist. Laparoscopy with chromotubation may be necessary to confirm and delineate Mullerian anomalies [27].

Recently, the advent of 3D ultrasound has added a new investigative tool for the evaluation of Mullerian anomalies. It has been shown to be highly accurate in the diagnosis of uterine malformations; with a sensitivity of 98–100 % and specificity of 100 % [28]. There are limited studies that accurately compare MRI with 3D ultrasound in the diagnosis and classification of uterine anomalies, but 3D ultrasound has the possibility of emerging as the new standard as it appears to be more sensitive and specific than MRI in the categorization of specific types of Mullerian duct anomalies; however, results may vary depending on the expertise and experience of the sonographer.

Prior to the introduction of magnetic resonance imaging (MRI)—ultrasound, hysterosalpingography, laparoscopy, and laparotomy were used in diagnosing and evaluating Mullerian anomalies [21]. However, a review of the literature found that ultrasound might only be 26 % sensitive at detecting this anomaly [3]. Disadvantages of hysterosalpingography include limited use in the very young, virginal patient; exposure of the patient to contrast material and radiation; and the inability to accurately differentiate uterine subtypes [19]. The disadvantages of laparoscopy and laparotomy are their invasiveness and inherent surgical risks.

The use of MRI for the diagnosis of Mullerian anomalies remains the gold standard, but may be second to 3D ultrasound in the future.

Treatment

Extirpation of uterine horns is the standard treatment in cases of noncommunicating or obstructing uterine horns.

There are three reasons for excision of rudimentary uterine horns: removing the cause of dysmenorrhea; preventing possible endometriosis caused by transtubal menstrual reflux; and avoiding rudimentary horn pregnancy implantation; all with the goal of alleviation of symptoms and conserving and optimizing fertility [20].

Prior to elective surgical repair, the initial management may include menstrual suppression with hormonal therapy such as oral contraceptive pills or depot medroxyprogesterone acetate. Gonadotropin-releasing hormone agonists (GnRH) have been used for suppression to allow time for additional imaging and the development of a surgical plan when necessary [23]. GnRH

analogues have been used for preoperative suppression if severe endometriosis is suspected [29].

Given the high incidence of concomitant rental anomalies (31–100 %), most clinicians propose performing renal imaging prior to the surgery [3, 5, 30]. An intravenous urogram may delineate the course and number of ureters [15].

Additional preoperative considerations should be given to the degree of myometrial connection between the uterine horns (Fig. 11.10) to be aware of the possible need for laparoscopic suture repair of the residual myometrial defect following resection of the noncommunicating rudimentary horn (Fig. 11.11).

Other preoperative considerations include noting the presence of a uterine mass, abnormalities in vaginal or cervical anatomy, the length of symptoms, and the history of any prior abdominal surgery [15]. These factors may help prepare the surgical team for the difficulty of the case.

While in the past excision of uterine horns were accomplished via a laparotomy, the current standard of care is a laparoscopic surgical approach. There have been several series highlighting the use of laparoscopy [15, 23, 24, 31–33]. This shift away from laparotomy is similar to the trend toward minimally invasive surgery for other gynecologic procedures. The benefits of minimally invasive surgery include a decreased length of hospital stay, a quicker return to activities of daily living, and improved cosmesis [23].

The primary principle for surgical resection of a uterine horn is to completely delineate the Mullerian structures and their connections. Initially, it may be necessary to confirm the non-

a

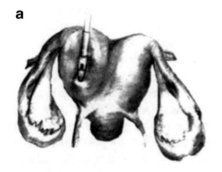

b

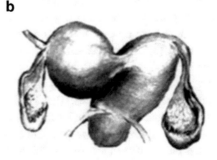

Fig. 11.10 Anatomical attachment between rudimentary horn and the hemiuterus. Rudimentary horn broadly attached to the unicornuate uterus (**a**) and minimally con-nected by a fibrous band (**b**). (Fedele L, Dorta M, Brioschi D et al. Magnetic resonance evaluation of double uteri. Obstet Gynecol 1980;74:844-847)

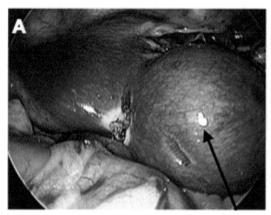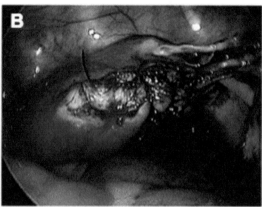

Fig. 11.11 (**a**) Laparoscopic transaction of functional, noncommunicating uterine horn and (**b**) suturing of myometrial defect in layers. (Spitzer RF, Kives S, Allen L. Case series of laparoscopically resected noncommunicating functional uterine horns. J Pediatr Adoles Gynecol 2009;22:e23-e28)

communicating side by performing chromotubation using methylene blue dye injected through the cervix and watching for efflux from the fallopian tube of the patent side, and a lack thereof from the obstructed side [23].

An assessment of the relative location of the horn to the unicornuate uterus should be completed to determine if they are separate, joined by a thin filmy band, or fused. When a fibrous band connects them, the primary blood supply to the rudimentary horn is from the ipsilateral uterine artery, and courses below the fibrous band, and is easy to coagulate or ligate [34].

However, when the rudimentary horn is firmly attached to the unicornuate uterus, the blood supply typically runs laterally to the unicornuate uterus and below the uterine horn, making hemostasis more difficult. In this situation, the rudimentary horn is likely to receive its blood supply from both the ipsilateral uterine artery and from the myometrial arcuate arteries of the contralateral uterine artery [35]. These vessels will require coagulation before dissection [20, 35].

The surgical steps of resection are similar to that of a laparoscopic hysterectomy (Fig. 11.12).

First, the round and utero-ovarian ligaments and the isthmic portion of the ipsilateral fallopian tube are transected on the side of the functional, noncommunicating horn. The broad ligament is incised enabling entrance into the retroperitoneal space to identify the ipsilateral ureter—remembering the

common associations of uterine anomalies with urologic anomalies. The vascular pedicle of the uterine horn may also be identified.

The uterovesical peritoneal fold is then incised and the bladder is reflected. Once this is accomplished, the uterine vessels for the noncommunicating horn are coagulated and transected. Attention can then be turned to transecting the horn from the remaining unicornuate uterus. This has been accomplished by a variety of techniques—a laparoscopic stapling device, bipolar cautery, endoscopic scissors, and the Harmonic scalpel (Ethicon EndoSurgery, Cincinnati, Ohio) [15, 24]. The ultrasonic energy scalpel has been reported to allow more accurate and easier dissection [36]. The ipsilateral fallopian tube should be removed along with the horn to decrease the risk of ectopic pregnancy [37].

The surgical challenge is to separate a densely fused horn from a rudimentary uterus. The dissection should err toward tissue preservation of the functional hemiuterus while at the same time excising all tissue associated with the noncommunicating horn, as even a small amount of residual cervical tissue may remain functional and cause gradual collection of menstrual blood and pain many years after the initial operation [38]. The use of hysteroscopic transillumination may be used to guide laparoscopic dissection in densely adherent rudimentary horns [39].

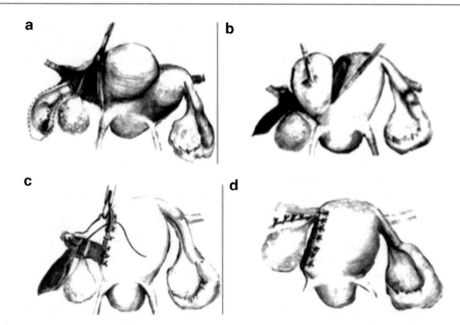

Fig. 11.12 Surgical steps for the laparoscopic removal of the rudimentary horn. The round ligament, fallopian tube, and utero-ovarian ligament are sectioned and the retroperitoneal space opened. (**a**). After coagulation and transection of the vascular pedicle, traction is applied and the horn is divided from the hemiuterus (**b**). The unicornuate uterus is sutured and the round ligament reattached (**c, d**). (Fedele L, Dorta M, Brioschi D et al. Magnetic resonance evaluation of double uteri. Obstet Gynecol 1980;74:844-847)

When there is significant fusion of the rudimentary horn to the unicornuate uterus at the cervical level, the use of thermocoagulation at the lower end of the rudimentary horn may help coagulate any remaining functional cervical tissue and prevent recurrences [38].

The specimen may be morcellated and removed from the abdomen. However, in the event that the morcellator is not available, the surgeon may elect to remove the intact specimen via a mini-laparotomy incision.

Of note, power morcellation has come under recent scrutiny due to concern about the risk of intraperitoneal dissemination of malignant tissue and a subsequent reduction in patient's long-term survival. This has led to a safety communication from the U.S. Food and Drug Administration which outlines the contraindications for morcellation use; specifically in peri- or postmenopausal women with fibroids, in women who are candidates for en bloc tissue removal, or in cases in which the tissue to be morcellated is known or suspected to contain malignancy [40].

The American Congress of Obstetricians and Gynecologists (ACOG) highlights that power morcellation is a well-established surgical technique, and without it, some patients would be ineligible for minimally invasive gynecologic surgery [41]. ACOG notes that with any surgical procedure appropriate preoperative evaluation, a discussion on the risks, benefits, and alternative treatment options, and obtaining informed consent is paramount.

While the risk of occult malignancy in premenopausal patients with noncommunicating uterine horns is low, there have been reports of disseminated tissue fragments implanting on organs in the abdominal cavity, with the potential for peritonitis, intra-abdominal abscesses, intestinal obstruction, or iatrogenic endometriosis or adenomyosis in patients without prior evidence of such conditions [42–45].

The authors maintain that with appropriate preoperative patient counseling and informed consent, power morcellation will continue to be a valuable tool in the resection of noncommunicating uterine horns. In cases in which the patient and surgeon feel the risks of power morcellation outweigh the benefits, the resected uterine horn may be removed from the abdomen via a mini-laparotomy.

Chromotubation may be used to evaluate for evidence of a myometrial defect at the site of the resection. In the event that one is noted, this should be closed in layers using a similar technique as that of a laparoscopic myomectomy. Robotic-assisted laparoscopy has been reported to improve visualization and ease of sewing defects in layers and may be a useful tool [46].

A recent review of long-term follow-up of patients who have undergone laparoscopic removal of noncommunicating rudimentary uterine horns revealed that complications from inadequate resection may occur as late as 6 years from the initial surgery. Three of 29 patients, who were followed for 10 years after their resection, had recurrent blood filled masses at the site of previous procedures requiring repeat surgical procedures for excision, thus highlighting the complexity of these cases and the importance of long-term evaluation [38].

There is a paucity of data on the rates of adhesions post-laparoscopic uterine horn resection; however, the data from laparoscopic myomectomies has shown lower rates of adhesion formation for laparoscopic techniques than open myomectomies [47]. Additionally, laparoscopic closure of uterine defects has been noted to be feasible and safe.

In cases of non-separated, noncommunicating horns, hysteroscopic resection of the midline septum with drainage of the hematometra and ablation of the endometrial tissue has been reported; but these techniques are not recommended due to the possibility of pregnancy implantation into the rudimentary horn from the contralateral side. These pregnancies have an increased risk of placenta accreta and uterine rupture [48–50].

El Saman has reported successful canalization of a noncommunicating uterine horn by horn-vaginal anastomosis without any dissection of the lower pole of the horn or vaginal apex [51]. This was performed in the case of a hypoplastic communicating horn and a well-developed but noncommunicating horn. The goal in this case was to allow the patient some reproductive function. Postoperatively, stenosis of the vaginal opening occurred and a repeat surgical procedure was required to place a vaginal-horn stent that remained in place to provide a connection and preserve menstrual egress. After a 4-month placement, the stent was removed and the patient was followed for 1 year. At the time of the report, the patient had 15 consecutive normal menstrual cycles. There are a few cases of pregnancies in cases of cervical atresia that support this management; however, due to risk of an ascending infection, recurrent obstruction, sepsis and potential death, some may advocate removal of isolated functioning uterine structures associated with cervical agenesis [52–57].

Metroplasty procedures have been described in the treatment of subseptate, septate, or bicornuate uteri. While this may be possible in fused cases of noncommunicating rudimentary horns, such procedures may not be possible if the rudimentary horn is separate from the other uterine horn. Furthermore, if there is a high degree of fusion between the uterine horns, dissection through the myometrium becomes necessary and the possibility of postsurgical stenosis is significant [15]. Lastly, by leaving the rudimentary horn in situ after a metroplasty procedure, the possibility of a pregnancy implanting in the smaller horn and a subsequent uterine rupture exists.

Impact on Fertility and Reproduction

Patients with noncommunicating uterine horns that contain functional endometrium are at an increased risk of ectopic pregnancy, hematosalpinx, endometriosis, and endometriomas secondary to retrograde menstruation. Adolescents with congenital obstructing Mullerian anomalies may have stage III or IV endometriosis even in early adolescence [58]. Resolution of the endometriosis after correction of the obstruction has been reported in the literature [59]; however, this may not always be the case, as other series have shown persistent disease after a relieved obstruction [60].

Rudimentary horn pregnancy occurs in 1 in 76,000 pregnancies [4]. The explanation of the pregnancy mechanism provided in the literature is the intraperitoneal transmigration of sperm or fertilized ova to the noncommunicating uterine horn. In the case of segregated twin pregnancy in noncommunicating hemiuteri, the explanation provided has been that multiple ovulation occurred and either sperm or a fertilized ovum transmigrated into the rudimentary horn, at the same that a second fertilized ovum implanted in the contralateral unicornuate horn [4]. Intraperitoneal sperm transmigration has been postulated to occur approximately 50 % of the time effecting spontaneous human pregnancies [37].

A 100-year (1900–1999) review of 588 cases of rudimentary uterine horn pregnancies revealed that 30 % of the gestations progressed to term or beyond. Fifty percent of the pregnant uterine horns ruptured—with 80 % of ruptures occurring before the third trimester. The overall survival rate of a singleton pregnancy in a rudimentary uterine horn was noted to be 6.1 %, with 46 % of the pregnancies reaching term [61].

This same series noted an overall maternal mortality rate of 1.2 % over the past 50 years. The majority of maternal deaths (80 %) were due to uterine rupture with 25 % occurring in the first trimester, 50 % in the second trimester, and 25 % in the third trimester.

Because of the risk of rupture, the traditional management of rudimentary horn pregnancies has been immediate surgical removal of the rudimentary horn with the pregnancy in situ regardless of gestational age. However, with improvements in fetal and maternal survival over the past 50 years and improvements in antenatal monitoring, rudimentary horn pregnancies recognized during the latter part of the second trimester may be managed conservatively. This decision should be based on whether or not there is evidence of a uniformly thick-walled uterine horn based on pelvic imaging studies. In theses cases, counseling must include discussions on how to balance the goal of prolonging the gestation to maximize chances of newborn survival, while minimizing risks of uterine rupture to both the fetus and the mother. Serial ultrasonography

should be undertaken to monitor the uterine wall thickness, as these congenitally abnormal uteri tend to become very thin as the pregnancies advance [61]. An estimated uterine wall thickness of less than 5 mm is related to an increased risk of impending hemiuterine rupture [62, 63].

In Nahum's review of 588 rudimentary horn pregnancies, 30 % continued to term or beyond [61], demonstrating in some properly selected and monitored patients there can be a good outcome. However, the best management is to deliver the pregnancy at the earliest possible time after an opportunity for fetal lung maturity. Each case should be managed individually, and with informed patient consent regarding the risks of maternal and fetal outcomes.

Nahum completed a review of the factors associated with maternal and fetal outcomes of rudimentary horn pregnancies and found that the only single factor that positively correlated with both decreasing mortality ($r=0.51$) and increasing neonatal survival ($r=0.74$) is earlier delivery of pregnancy. As a result, a reasonable management plan is an elective cesarean section with possible hemihysterectomy considered at either 28 completed weeks of gestation, when the estimated fetal weight exceeds 1000 g, or when the hemiuterine wall is diminished or less than 5 mm in any aspect on obstetric imaging, whichever clinical situation occurs first [61]. The recommended mode of delivery of a uterine horn pregnancy is cesarean section, with avoidance of uterine contractions during labor that may increase the risk of uterine horn rupture. Nahum's review quotes average gestational age and weight of newborn survivors to be 32 weeks and 1770 g, respectively, with a recent estimate of maternal mortality of less than 0.5 % despite rupture rates of 50 %.

The muscle of the horn is thin and in many cases the placentation is pathological, with placenta accreta, increta, and percreta occurring in some cases. These situations have an increased risk of postpartum hemorrhage due to the abnormal placental invasion of the myometrium and the underdeveloped musculature of rudimentary horns.

A prevailing theme is that the outcome of these pregnancies is poor [64, 65]—with an increased risk of miscarriage, ectopic pregnancy, preterm labor, malpresentation [1, 66, 67], intrauterine growth restriction and intrauterine fetal death [3]. In addition, failed terminations of pregnancy have been reported [68–70].

Heterotopic pregnancy in unicornuate uteri with rudimentary horns has a probability of 1 in 43,000,000 gestations [3], but has been reported in the literature [4, 71, 72]. Twin pregnancy in a unicornuate uterus has an incidence of 5 % and a reported overall survival rate of 2.4 % [61].

The prognosis of intrauterine pregnancy is not significantly impaired when located in the unicornuate uterus, although there is a risk of intrauterine growth restriction, premature labor and delivery, breech presentation, and a higher number of cesarean sections [1]. Heinonen has noted an increase in pregnancy-induced hypertension in patients with a unicornuate pregnancy and a single kidney [1].

Limited data are available regarding future fertility in patients in whom excision of rudimentary horns have been undertaken [73].

Conclusions

Noncommunicating rudimentary uterine horns are common findings associated with unicornuate uteri. When the horn has functional endometrium, patients typically present in the post-menarchal period with pain symptoms secondary to the obstruction. The use of MRI to correctly diagnose the anomaly is crucial—as several other entities may be confused as a noncommunicating rudimentary horn. Once a patient is diagnosed with an obstructed horn, surgical intervention is indicated. The horn is resected most often via minimally invasive techniques. Treatment goals are twofold—relief of pain symptoms and preservation of optimal fertility. Patients with noncommunicating uterine horns that contain functional endometrium are at an increased risk endometriosis, endometriomas, hematosalpinx, and poor pregnancy outcomes. We are optimistic that with continued advances in and increased utilization of 3D ultrasound, this particular anomaly may be diagnosed without delay—thus minimizing the effect of pain, infertility, and pregnancy morbidities for our patients.

References

1. Heinonen P. Unicornuate uterus and rudimentary horn. Fertil Steril. 1997;68:224–30.
2. Naham GG. Uterine anomalies: how common are they, and what is there distribution among subtypes? J Reprod Med. 1998;43:877–87.
3. Jayasinghe Y, Rane A, Stalewski H, et al. The presentation and early diagnosis of the rudimentary uterine horn. Obstet Gynecol. 2005;105:1456–67.
4. Nahum G. Rudimentary horn pregnancy: case report on surviving twins delivered 8 days apart. J Reprod Med. 1997;42:525–32.
5. Silber CG, Magness RL, Farber M. Duplication of the uterus with a non-communicating functioning uterine horn. Mt Sinai J Med. 1990;57:374–7.
6. Davis AJ, Hostetler B, Reindollar RH. Canalization failure of the mullerian tract. Fertil Steril. 1992; 58:826–8.
7. Anderson CW. A theory which explains uterine anomalies, dextroversion and dextrorotation, and other phenomena. Urol Cut Rev. 1943;46:556–8.
8. Acien P, Acien M, Fernandez F, et al. The cavitated accessory uterine mass: a mullerian anomaly in women with an otherwise normal uterus. Obstet Gynecol. 2010;116:1101–9.
9. Potter DA, Schenken RS. Noncommunicating accessory uterine cavity. Fertil Steril. 1998;70:1165–6.
10. Dogen E, Gode F, Saatli B, Secil M. Juvenile cystic adenomyosis mimicking uterine malformation: a case report. Arch Gynecol Obstet. 2008;278:593–5.
11. Tok CH, Bux SI, Mohammed SI, et al. Degenerated uterine fibroid mimicking hydrometra: fallacy in CT. Biomed Imaging Interv J. 2006;2(4):e42.1–4.
12. Gaied F, Quiros-Calinoiu E, Emil S. Laparoscopic excision of a rudimentary uterine horn in a child. J Pediatr Surg. 2011;46:411–4.
13. Yeko TR, Parsons AK, Marshall R, Maroulis G. Laparoscopic removal of mullerian remnants in a woman with congenital absence of the vagina. Fertil Steril. 1992;57:218–20.
14. Semmens JP. Congenital anomalies of female genital tract. Functional classification based on review of 56 personal cases. Obstet Gynecol. 1962;19:328–50.
15. Strawbridge LC, Crouch NS, Cutner AS, Creighton SM. Obstructive mullerian anomalies and modern laparoscopic management. J Pediatr Adolesc Gynecol. 2007;20:195–200.
16. Heinonen PK. Clinical implications of the unicornuate uterus with rudimentary horn. Int J Gynaecol Obstet. 1983;21:145–50.
17. Edmonds DK. Treatment of anomalies of the reproductive tract. In: Sanfilippo JS, Lara-Torre E, Edmonds DK, et al., editors. Clinical pediatric and adolescent gynecology. New York: Informa Healthcare USA; 2009. p. 393.
18. Kamio M, Nagata T, Yamasaki H, Yoshinaga M, Douchi T. Inguinal hernia containing functioning, rudimentary uterine horn and endometriosis. Obstet Gynecol. 2009;113:563–6.

19. Pellerito JS, McCarthy SM, Doyle MB, Glickman MG, DeCherney AH. Diagnosis of uterine anomalies: relative accuracy of MR imaging, endovaginal sonography, and hysterosalpinography. Radiology. 1992;183:795–800.
20. Fedele L, Dorta M, Brioschi D, et al. Magnetic resonance evaluation of double uteri. Obstet Gynecol. 1980;74:844–7.
21. Marten K, Vosshenrich R, Funke M, Obenauer S, Baum F, Grabbe E. MRI in the evaluation of mullerian duct anomalies. J Clin Imaging. 2003;27:346–50.
22. Carbognin G, Guarise A, Minelli L, Vitale I, Malago R, Zamboni G. Pelvic endometriosis: US and MRI features. Abdom Imaging. 2004;29:609–18.
23. Spitzer RF, Kives S, Allen L. Case series of laparoscopically resected noncommunicating functional uterine horns. J Pediatr Adolesc Gynecol. 2009;22:e23–8.
24. Dietrich JE, Young AE, Young RL. Resection of a non-communicating uterine horn with use of the harmonic scalpel. J Pediatr Adolesc Gynecol. 2004;17:407–9.
25. Economy KE, Barnewolt C, Laufer MR. A comparison of MRI and laparoscopy in detecting pelvic structures in cases of vaginal agenesis. J Pediatr Adolesc Gynecol. 2002;15:101–4.
26. Zurawin RK, Dietrich JE, Heard MJ, et al. Didelphic uterus and obstructed hemivagina with renal agenesis: case report and review of the literature. J Pediatr Adolesc Gynecol. 2004;17:137–41.
27. Devine K, McCluskey T, Henne M, et al. Is magnetic resonance imaging sufficient to diagnose a rudimentary uterine horn: a case report and review of the literature. J Minim Invasive Surg. 2013;20:533–6.
28. Deutch TD, Abuhamad AZ. The role of 3-dimensional ultrasonography and magnetic resonance imaging in the diagnosis of mullerian duct anomalies. J Ultrasound Med. 2008;27:413–23.
29. Canis M, Wattiez A, Pouly JL, et al. Laparoscopic management of unicornuate uterus with rudimentary horn and unilateral extensive endometriosis: case report. Hum Reprod. 1990;5:819–20.
30. Buttram Jr VC, Gibbons WE. Mullerian anomalies: a proposed classification (an analysis of 144 cases). Fertil Steril. 1979;32:40–6.
31. Tanaka Y, Asada H, Uchida H, et al. Case of iatrogenic dysmenorrhea in non-communicating rudimentary uterine horn and its laparoscopic resection. J Obstet Gynaecol Res. 2005;31:242–6.
32. Fedele L, Bianchi S, Zanconato G, et al. Laparoscopic removal of the cavitated noncommunicating rudimentary uterine horn: surgical aspects in 10 cases. Fertil Steril. 2005;83:432–6.
33. Takeuchi H, Sato Y, Shimanuki H, et al. Accurate preoperative diagnosis and laparoscopic removal of the cavitated non-communicated uterine horn for obstructive mullerian anomalies. J Obstet Gynaecol Res. 2006;32:74–9.
34. Falcone T, Hemmings R, Khalife S. Laparoscopic management of a unicornuate uterus with a rudimentary horn. J Gynecol Surg. 1995;11:105–7.
35. Perrotin F, Bertrand J, Body G. Laparoscopic surgery of unicornuate uterus with rudimentary uterine horn. Hum Reprod. 1999;14:931–3.
36. Creighton SM, Minto CL, Cutner AS. Use of the ultrasonically activated scalpel in laparoscopic resection of a noncommunicating rudimentary horn. Gynaecol Endosc. 2009;9:327–9.
37. Nahum G, Stanislaw H, McMahon C. Preventing ectopic pregnancies: how often does transperitoneal transmigration of sperm occur in effecting human pregnancy? BJOG. 2004;111:706–14.
38. Nakhal RS, Cutner AS, Hall-Craggs M, et al. Remnant functioning cervical tissue after laparoscopic removal of cavitated non-communicating rudimentary uterine horn. J Minim Invas Gynecol. 2012;19:768–71.
39. Nazhat F, Nazhat C, Bess O, et al. Laparoscopic amputation of a noncommunicating rudimentary horn after a hysteroscopic diagnosis: a case study. Surg Laparosc Endosc. 1994;4(2):155–6.
40. Food and Drug Administration. Updated laparoscopic uterine power morcellation in hysterectomy and myomectomy: FDA safety communication. FDA; 2014. Available at: http://www.fda.gov/MedicalDevices/Safety/AlertsandNotices/ucm424443.htm. Retrieved 18 March 2015.
41. The American Congress of Obstetricians and Gynecologists. Power morcellation and occult malignancy in gynecologic surgery: a special report. ACOG; 2014. Available at: http://acog.org/Resources-And-Publications/Task-Force-and-Work-Group-Reports/Power-Morcellation-and-Occult-Malignancy-in-Gynecologic-Surgery. Retrieved 18 March 2015.
42. Milad MP, Milad EA. Laparoscopic morcellator-related complications. J Minim Invasive Gynecol. 2014;21:486–91.
43. Sepilian V, Della Badia C. Iatrogenic endometriosis caused by uterine morcellation during a supracervical hysterectomy. Obstet Gynecol. 2003;102:1125–7.
44. Donnez O, Squifflet J, Leconte I, et al. Posthysterectomy pelvic adenomyotic masses observed in 8 cases out of a series of 1405 laparoscopic subtotal hysterectomies. J Minim Invasive Gynecol. 2007;14(2):156–60.
45. American Association of Gynecologic Laparoscopists (AAGL). Morcellation during uterine tissue extraction. AAGL; 2014. Available at: http://www.aagl.org/wp-content/uploads/2014/05/Tissue_Extraction_TFR.pdf. Retrieved 18 March 2015.
46. Dietrich JE, Millar DM, Quint EH. Obstructive reproductive tract anomalies. J Pediatr Adolesc Gynecol. 2014;27:396–402.
47. Hurst BS, Matthews ML, Marshburn PB. Laparoscopic myomectomy for symptomatic uterine myomas. Fertil Steril. 2005;83:1–23.
48. von Eye CH, Villodre LC, Reis R, et al. Conservative treatment of a noncommunicating rudimentary uterine horn. Acta Obstet Gynecol Scand. 2001;80:668.
49. Hucke J, DeBruyne F, Campo RL, et al. Hysteroscopic treatment of congenital uterine malformations

causing hematometra: a report of three cases. Fertil Steril. 1992;58:823–5.

50. Perino A, Chianchiano H, Simonaro C, et al. Endoscopic management of a case of complete septate uterus with unilateral haematometra. Hum Reprod. 1995;10:2171–3.

51. El Saman AM, Habib DM, Othman ER, et al. Successful canalization of a non-communicating uterine horn by horn-vaginal anastomosis: preliminary findings of a novel approach for an unclassified anomaly. J Pediatr Surg. 2011;46:1464–8.

52. Farber M, Marchant DJ. Reconstructive surgery for congenital atresia of the uterine cervix. Fertil Steril. 1976;27:1277–82.

53. Cukier J, Batzofin JH, Stanley Conner J, et al. Genital tract reconstruction in a patient with congenital absence of the vagina and hypoplasia of the cervix. Obstet Gynecol. 1986;68:32S–6.

54. Fujimoto VY, Heath Miller J, Klein NA, et al. Congenital cervical atresia: report of seven cases and review of the literature. Am J Obstet Gynecol. 1997;177:1419–25.

55. Deffarges JV, Haddad B, Musset R, et al. Uterovaginal anastomosis in women with uterine cervix atresia: long-term follow-up and reproductive performance. A study of 18 cases. Hum Reprod. 2001; 16:1722–5.

56. Bugmann P, Amaudruz M, Hanquinet S, et al. Uterocervicoplasty with a bladder mucosa layer for the treatment of complete cervical agenesis. Fertil Steril. 2002;77:831–5.

57. Creighton SM, Davies MC, Cutner A. Laparoscopic management of cervical agenesis. Fertil Steril. 2006;85:1510.e13–15.

58. Laufer MR. Gynecologic pain: dysmenorrhea, acute and chronic pelvic pain, endometriosis, and premenstrual syndrome. In: Emans SJ, Laufer MR, editors. Pediatric and adolescent gynecology. 6th ed. Philadelphia: Lippincott Williams & Wilkins; 2012. p. 258.

59. Sanfilippo JS, Wakim NG, Schikler KN, et al. Endometriosis in association with uterine anomaly. Am J Obstet Gynecol. 1986;154:39–43.

60. Silveira SA, Laufer MR. Persistence of endometriosis after correction of an obstructed reproductive tract anomaly. J Pediatr Adolesc Gynecol. 2013;26:e93–4.

61. Nahum GG. Rudimentary uterine horn pregnancy: the 20th-century worldwide experience of 588 cases. J Reprod Med. 2002;47:151–63.

62. Achiron R, Tadmor O, Kamar R, et al. Pre-rupture ultrasound diagnosis of interstitial and rudimentary uterine horn pregnancy in the second trimester. J Reprod Med. 1992;37:89–92.

63. Gagnon AL, Galerneau F, Williams K. Twin pregnancy in the rudimentary horn of a bicornuate uterus associated with renal agenesis. Am J Obstet Gynecol. 1941;42:534–6.

64. Donderwinkel PF, Dorr JP, Willemsen WN. The unicornuate uterus: clinical implications. Eur J Obstet Gynecol Reprod Biol. 1992;47:135–9.

65. Raga F, Bauset C, Remohi J, et al. Reproductive impact of congenital mullerian anomalies. Hum Reprod. 1997;12:2277–81.

66. Soundararajan V, Rai J. Laparoscopic removal of a rudimentary uterine horn during pregnancy: a case report. J Reprod Med. 2000;45:599–602.

67. Heinonen P, Saarikoski S, Pystynen P. Reproductive performance of women with uterine anomalies. Acta Obstet Gynecol Scand. 1982;61:157–62.

68. Rolen AC, Choquette AJ, Semmens JP. Rudimentary uterine horn: obstetric and gynecologic implications. Obstet Gynecol. 1966;27:806–13.

69. Ghosh N. Pregnancy in the rudimentary horn of a bicornuate uterus. Int Surg. 1966;46:567–72.

70. Ural SH, Artal R. Third-trimester rudimentary horn pregnancy: a case report. J Reprod Med. 1998;43:919–21.

71. Pongsuthirak P, Tongsong T, Srisomboon J. Rupture of a noncommunicating rudimentary uterine horn pregnancy with a combined intrauterine pregnancy. Int J Gynecol Obstet. 1993;41:185–7.

72. Sahakian V. Rupture of a rudimentary horn pregnancy with a combined intrauterine pregnancy: a case report. J Reprod Med. 1992;37:283–4.

73. Adolph AJ, Gilliland GB. Fertility following laparoscopic removal of rudimentary horn with an ectopic pregnancy. J Obstet Gynaecol Can. 2002;24:575–6.

Obstructed Hemivagina

12

Nigel Pereira and Samantha M. Pfeifer

Congenital obstructive malformations of the female reproductive tract constitute of a group structural malformations arising from the abnormal development of the Müllerian ducts. Obstructed hemivagina in association with a double uterus and renal anomaly has been described as early as 1922 [1]. Since then, this anomaly has been described in the literature associated with several different names: double uterus with obstructed hemivagina and ipsilateral renal agenesis [2], obstructed hemivagina and ipsilateral renal anomaly (OHVIRA) syndrome [3], and Herlyn-Werner-Wunderlich syndrome [4].

Incidence

It is difficult to accurately estimate the true incidence of obstructive Müllerian duct malformations in the general population, as most data regarding the condition arise from studies involving patients with reproductive problems [5]. Furthermore, accurate assessment of uterine anatomy and morphology are lacking in such studies [5]. Despite these limitations, the overall incidence of obstructive Müllerian duct malformations is thought to range from 0.1 to 3.8 % [6].

N. Pereira, M.D. (✉) • S.M. Pfeifer, M.D.
Weill Cornell Medical College, New York, NY
10021, USA
e-mail: nip9060@med.cornell.edu

Obstructed hemivagina is typically associated with a uterus didelphys or complete septate uterus as these conditions are often associated with a longitudinal vaginal septum [8] (Fig. 12.1). Purslow first described the combination of obstructed hemivagina and uterus didelphys in 1922 [1]. Since then, over 250 cases have been reported in the medical literature [7]. The combination of an obstructed hemivagina, uterus didelphys, and ipsilateral renal agenesis was first reported as a syndrome in 1971 [9] with an incidence ranging from 1 in 2000 to 1 in 28,000 [10]. Variability of the anatomic structures involved in this syndrome is well known [2]. While most reports have described the uterine anomaly as uterus didelphys, septate, and bicornuate uterus has also been reported [2, 11, 12]. Unilateral obstruction associated with this syndrome is mainly vaginal, but cervical obstruction has been occasionally described [2, 11, 12]. Reports of dysplastic or duplicated kidneys may also be found associated with the syndrome [2, 12].

The anomaly uterus didelphys or septate uterus with obstructed hemivagina is not captured or described by the AFS Classification system as this classification does not describe vaginal anomalies [13]. The newer classification systems do consider vaginal, cervical, and uterine anomalies and are able to adequately categorize and describe these anomalies [14–16].

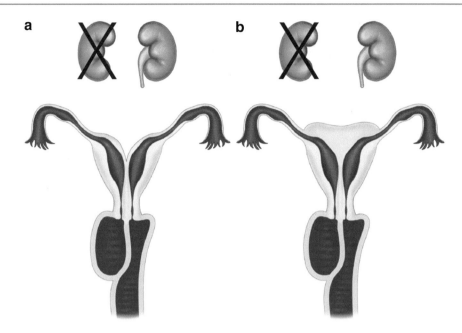

Fig. 12.1 (**a**) Uterus didelphys with obstructed right hemivagina. (**b**) Complete septate uterus with obstructed right hemivagina. Note renal agenesis ipsilateral to the obstruction in both cases

Etiology

Müllerian anomalies generally occur around the eighth week of gestation [17]. An isolated vaginal septum is thought to arise due to failed resorption of the uterovaginal septum [18]. However, the pathogenesis of the triad of uterine didelphys, obstructed hemivagina, and ipsilateral renal agenesis is more complex. The putative embryonic mechanism is likely due to a disruption in the development of the caudal portion of one mesonephric duct with secondary involvement of the ipsilateral Müllerian duct [2]. On the affected side, the mesonephric duct anomaly accounts for failure of regular ureteric budding and kidney differentiation, with consequent renal agenesis, as well as an abnormal location of ipsilateral Müllerian duct. This results in the failure of the abnormal Müllerian duct fuse with both its opposite counterpart and with the urogenital sinus, thereby creating a double uterus and cervico-vaginal obstruction [2, 11].

The double uterus described with this anomaly may have many configurations, which have been described in a series of 87 patients [2] (Fig. 12.2). The most common presentation is that of a uterus didelphys with two separate uterine horns occurring in 77 % of patients [2, 19]. The second most common variant in this series is a complete septate uterus with duplicated cervices, or septate bicollis occurring in 14 % of cases [2, 19] In another study, the incidence of obstructed hemivagina with uterus didelphys or a complete septate uterus was 57 % and 29 %, respectively [19]. Less common variants described include a bicornuate bicollis configuration, didelphic uterus with unilateral cervical atresia, and bicornuate uterus with septate cervix and obstructed hemivagina. With the uterus didelphys and complete septate variants, the right and left sides are separate and noncommunicating. The obstruction may be complete or partial. With complete obstruction presenting symptoms occur earlier. Partial obstruction involves a communication or microperforation between the obstructed hemivagina and normal vagina. In addition, there may be a communication occurring higher up in the reproductive tract such as within the cervix or uterine cavities [2, 10, 11] (Fig. 12.3).

Double uterus with obstructed hemivagina is seen in association with renal anomalies in 90–95 % of cases, with 5–10 % of patients having two normal kidneys [3, 11]. The most commonly reported renal anomaly seen is ipsilateral renal

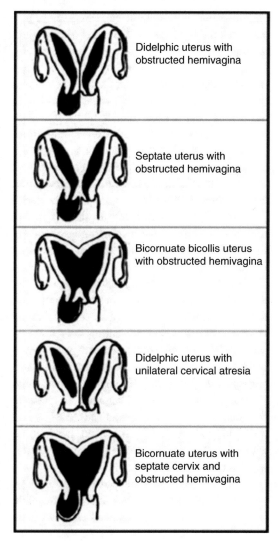

Didelphic uterus with obstructed hemivagina

Septate uterus with obstructed hemivagina

Bicornuate bicollis uterus with obstructed hemivagina

Didelphic uterus with unilateral cervical atresia

Bicornuate uterus with septate cervix and obstructed hemivagina

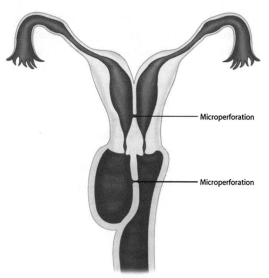

Fig. 12.3 Uterus didelphys with obstructed hemivagina depicting locations of microperforation

Fig. 12.2 Anatomic illustration and description of anatomic variants seen with double uterus and obstructed hemivagina. (*Fedele L, et al. Double uterus with obstructed hemivagina and ipsilateral renal agenesis: pelvic anatomic variants in 87 cases. Hum Reprod 2013;28(6):1580-3*)

agenesis occurring in approximately 95 % of patients. Other real anomalies reported include dysplastic kidney, duplicated ureter, and polycystic kidney. Right-sided obstruction with ipsilateral renal agenesis is seen more commonly than left-sided obstruction [20] with an incidence 62–77 % noted in the larger case series [4, 11, 19, 21]. In the largest systematic review of 138 patients, right-sided obstruction was noted in 65 % of the study population [11]. Similarly, in a series of 70 patients, right-sided predominance was noted in 62 % of

patients [4]. Several mechanisms have been proposed to account for this asymmetry. Differences in gene expression on either side of the embryo at various times during development can result in unequal sensitivity of paired structures to teratogens and adverse genetic influences during organogenesis. This may lead to differences in the lateral distribution of some birth defects [22]. It is also thought that the left side of the embryo has greater mitochondrial maturity compared to the right, resulting in higher energy reserves and lesser tissue damage [23]. The right side, is therefore, more susceptible to hypoxic damage than the left [24]. Despite these mechanisms, the actual cause for this asymmetry still remains elusive [11].

Differential Diagnosis

When evaluating a patient with suspected double uterus with obstructed hemivagina menses occur normally from the non-obstructed side. As menstruation appears to be occurring normally, dysmenorrhea and pain symptoms are often not addressed and may be attributed to "bad menstrual cramps," possible endometriosis or non-gynecologic causes. The challenge is to recognize the pain symptoms, which typically become increasingly severe over a short period of time, and consider a Müllerian anomaly in the differential diagnosis, especially if the adolescent has a known congenital renal agenesis. One must differentiate this condition from an obstructed uterine horn, which may have a similar presentation. Imaging studies such ultrasound and magnetic resonance imaging (MRI) will distinguish the location of the obstruction and will reveal the presence of cervix and hematocolpos in the setting of obstructed hemivagina. With uterus didelphys and obstructed hemivagina with microperforation, these patients typically present with regular menstruation, but complain of persistent vaginal spotting throughout the menstrual cycle or purulent vaginal discharge. This condition is often confused with abnormal uterine bleeding, vaginitis, or a sexually transmitted disease. Again imaging, preferably MRI, can define the anatomy and identify the uterine anomaly.

Diagnosis

The diagnosis of obstructed hemivagina is difficult due to its rarity, as well as its nonspecific signs and symptoms, and commonly a lack of consideration of a Müllerian anomaly in the differential diagnosis [25]. Patients usually remain asymptomatic until menarche [12], though rare presentations in the neonatal period have also been reported [26]. Symptoms usually become apparent within several months postmenarche and are described as progressively worsening abdominal pain or dysmenorrhea [12, 25]. Presenting symptoms occur as a result of a build up of menstrual fluid within the obstructed hemivagina and subsequently the uterus, fallopian tube, and abdominal cavity due to retrograde menstruation. These symptoms are often not recognized because menstruation occurs normally through the patent and non-affected side [3, 12]. As a result, the diagnosis is often delayed for months to years after menarche [4]. The most common presenting symptom at diagnosis is dysmenorrhea [4, 27] typically progressive, escalating, and severe eventually limiting the patient's ability to participate in normal activities. Other symptoms include abdominal pain, pelvic

or abdominal pressure, urinary frequency, urinary retention, constipation, and paravaginal mass [27].

In girls who have a communication between the obstructed and patent sides, symptoms typically include cyclic menstruation and dysmenorrhea, but with irregular and continuous spotting between periods reflecting a slow egress of the menstrual blood in the obstructed side through the microperforation and into the patent side [4, 27]. In addition, infection may develop in the obstructed side from ascending bacterial infection. If there is infection in the obstructed vaginal canal, there can be continuous, profuse, and malodorous purulent vaginal discharge. Frequently, this discharge is assumed to be vaginitis or a sexually transmitted disease, and the patient has undergone numerous courses of antibiotics without success, often over several months to years. The age and presenting symptoms of patients with obstructed hemivagina varies according to the degree of obstruction. In a retrospective study of 70 patients, mean age (±standard deviation) at diagnosis in patients with complete obstruction was 13.0 (±2.1) years while in patients with obstructed hemivagina with microperforation mean age at presentation was later 24.7 (±7.7) [4].

Delay in diagnosis can lead to the development of upper tract disease due to retrograde menstruation and development of endometriosis and adhesions [28, 29]. In one case series, common findings at laparoscopy in patients with double uterus with obstructed hemivagina included: endometriosis 37 %, hematosalpinx 22 %, pelvic adhesions 10 %, and 1 case of pysosalpinx [27]. These findings have been noted in other studies [3, 4]. These conditions are also correlated with development of abdominal pain and infertility. Therefore, the longer the delay in diagnosis, the greater the risk for development of these upper tract findings, and subsequent infertility.

Abdominal examination may reveal a tender suprapubic or abdominal mass [12]. Pelvic or rectal examination can be significant for a paravaginal cystic mass [12]. Often, pelvic examinations in adolescents or virginal females may be significantly limited and in some cases traumatic for the individual and not helpful in clarifying the diagnosis [6]. Radiologic imaging, therefore, plays an important role in the diagnosis. When double uterus with obstructed hemivagina is suspected, ultrasonography (US) can be performed initially to delineate abnormalities of the genitourinary tract [7]. US serves as an important tool in the detection of hematocolpos, which usually appears as a rounded, smooth-walled, hypoechoic mass with absent flow on Doppler imaging [6, 10]. However, to facilitate accurate diagnosis,

MRI should be performed. Compared to US, MRI provides more detailed information regarding uterine morphology and continuity with each vaginal canal, thereby facilitating the most appropriate treatment strategy [10] (Figs. 12.4 and 12.5). Three-dimensional ultrasound is helpful in distinguishing septate from bicornuate uterus, but may not be helpful in determining the specific anatomic defect or the level of the obstruction. Laparoscopic evaluation of pelvic anatomy should be considered when MRI is non-diagnostic

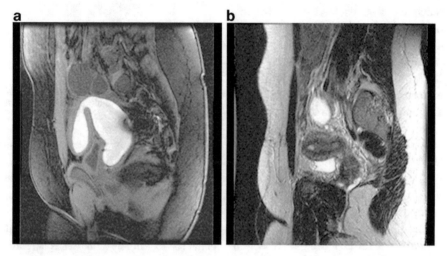

Fig. 12.4 (**a**) MRI showing hematocolpos with hematometra and well-defined cervical canal. (**b**) Normal uterine horn with normal endometrial cavity

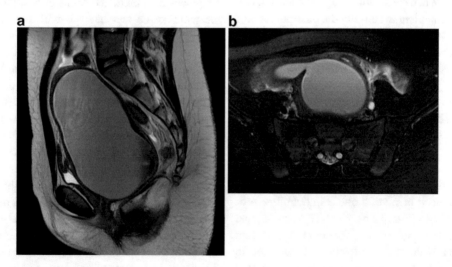

Fig. 12.5 (**a**) MRI showing large hematocolpos due to uterus didelphys with obstructed hemivagina. In this case, the obstruction is low as evidenced by close proximity to the symphysis. (**b**) Axial view MRI showing hematocolpos and right hematometra and well-defined and dilated cervix

or when an experienced radiologist is unavailable [2, 4, 6]. In general, computerized tomography is not helpful in delineating anatomy of Müllerian anomalies.

The presence of uterine didelphys and obstructed hemivagina is highly correlated with unilateral renal agenesis ipsilateral to the obstruction. Given the prevalence of fetal ultrasonography, unilateral renal agenesis is often diagnosed prior to birth. Therefore, increasing dysmenorrhea in a young adolescent with a history of renal agenesis should trigger an evaluation for uterine didelphys and obstructed hemivagina, which would facilitate early diagnosis.

It is important to clarify the specific uterine anomaly seen in association with the obstructed hemivagina so as to better counsel the patient regarding treatment options as well as future fertility and reproductive outcomes.

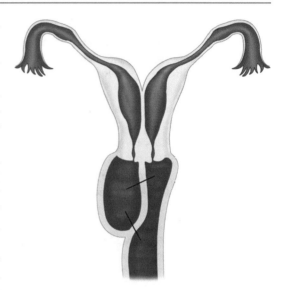

Fig. 12.6 Uterus didelphys with obstructed right hemivagina with location of resection site for resecting the vaginal septum

Treatment

There are several options to treat double uterus with obstructed hemivagina including primary resection, removal of the vagina and uterus on the obstructed side, and drainage techniques to acutely relieve symptoms of obstruction with subsequent hormonal suppression of menses to defer septum resection. When considering surgical management, it is also important to consider the maturity level of the patient and family dynamics. Social work and adolescent medicine specialists may be helpful in the discussion of treatment options.

Resection of Vaginal Septum and Marsupialization

Primary resection of the vaginal septum with marsupialization is considered the optimal approach as it involves a one-step definitive procedure [3, 4] (Fig. 12.6). Several observational studies have demonstrated that complete septum resection with marsupialization is superior to simple incision and drainage as this procedure is associated with a higher rate of re-occlusion and infection [6, 12, 18]. The approach to primary

resection of the vaginal septum and marsupialization depends on the size of the hematocolpos and the location of the obstruction. If the vaginal obstruction is at the level of the lower vaginal segment, then the hematocolpos is relatively large and runs parallel to the normal vaginal canal [6, 25]. In this situation, it is relatively easy to identify and resect a large segment of the septum thereby creating a large window between the patent and obstructed hemivaginas. The larger the window the less likely it will close and reocclude. If, however, the obstruction is high in the vaginal canal, then the hematocolpos is smaller and the area of septum that can be resected is also small and therefore more likely to re-occlude. It can also be more difficult to identify the smaller hematocolpos at the time of surgery. Techniques that facilitate identifying the hematocolpos include palpation, insertion of 19G needle with syringe to aspirate and confirm the presence of menstrual blood and transabdominal ultrasound guidance [6, 18], placement of probe through the uterine fundus ipsilateral to the obstruction and passing it through the cervix to tent the lower edge of the obstructed vagina (similar to what is done with transverse vaginal septum [30]), and hydrodissection of the plane in between the hemivaginal septum and the cervix

[25]. Once the hematocolpos is identified, then the septum can be entered at the needle insertion site using a bovie or knife. A long clamp with narrow tip can then be used to further enlarge the opening and allow drainage of the hematocolpos. Following drainage, the septum can be palpated and resected using scissors/knife or cautery (bovie, ligasure). The septum can be very thick and vascular and suture ligature, cautery or vessel sealing techniques are helpful to control bleeding during marsupialization. In addition, the rectum and bladder are extremely close to the area of septum resection and after decompression of a hematocolpos the anatomy may not be distinct. Frequent rectal exams and cystoscopy can decrease the risk of, or identify, bowel and bladder injury.

Histologic evaluation of the resected vaginal septum in the obstructed side may reveal different histology then the typical expected squamous epithelium. Changes including columnar epithelium with glandular crypts of cervical type and adenosis have been reported [3, 21]. Long-term follow-up shows reversion to normal squamous epithelium over time [21].

Transvaginal septum resection using traditional specula or retractors may not be feasible in pediatric patients or patients who wish to preserve hymenal integrity. In such cases, resection of a vaginal septum can be undertaken using vaginoscopy [25, 31–34].

The risk of re-occlusion following resection has been reported to be approximately 5–24 % [3, 15, 35]. To reduce the risk of re-occlusion the resected portion of the vaginal septum should be as large as possible and constriction of the vaginal opening should be avoided if sutures are used for hemostasis. Placement of a vaginal dilator postoperatively to prevent re-occlusion is usually not indicated with this procedure.

The use of simultaneous laparoscopy at the time of vaginal septum resection for double uterus with obstructed hemivagina has been advocated [27]. However, others have recommended that routine laparoscopy at the time of vaginal septum resection is not indicated [3]. The concern with any obstructed Müllerian anomaly is retrograde menstruation and associated development of endometriosis that may lead subsequent issues of pain, adhesions, and infertility. However, the natural history of endometriosis that develops due to an obstructed Müllerian anomaly is not well understood. Spontaneous resolution of endometriosis in the setting of treatment of an obstructed hemivagina has been described [21, 36]; however, there are no large long-term studies evaluating this issue. When there is evidence of a hematosalpinx or ovarian endometrioma caused by an obstructed Müllerian anomaly, laparoscopy is recommended to surgically treat as these conditions do not resolve. The decision to perform simultaneous laparoscopy should therefore be based on the presence of hematosalpinx, ovarian endometrioma, severity of symptoms suggesting severe adhesive disease or endometriosis, interval between menarche and diagnosis, or need to confirm the diagnosis or anatomy.

When caring for a patient with obstructed hemivagina associated with a complete septate uterus, it is not advisable to resect the uterine septum at the same time. With distention of the endometrial cavity on the obstructed side, there is distortion of the anatomy and resecting the uterine septum may be more challenging increasing the risk of damage to the uterus with subsequent impact on reproductive function. Furthermore, although resection of a uterine septum may reduce miscarriage risk in some individuals, there are no data to recommend routine resection of a complete uterine septum in an asymptomatic individual. Individuals with complete septate uterus may have normal reproductive function.

Hemihysterectomy with Ipsilateral Hemicolpectomy

Hemihysterectomy with ipsilateral hemicolpectomy has been performed to treat double uterus with obstructed hemivagina [27] (Fig. 12.7). The vaginal tissue on the obstructed side must be removed with the uterus. If the vaginal mucosa is not removed, there is risk of development of a closed cavity lined with vaginal mucosa that may subsequently enlarge with vaginal secretions and

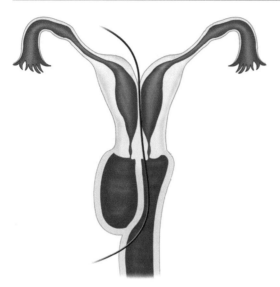

Fig. 12.7 Uterus didelphys with obstructed right hemivagina depicting resection of right uterine horn and obstructed hemivagina

cause pain. This procedure is more invasive than vaginal septum resection, involving either laparoscopy or laparotomy and extensive dissection. This procedure should probably be reserved for those cases where a safe vaginoplasty is difficult such as in the cases where the obstructed hemivagina is narrow, small, high, distant from the patent vagina, recurrent vaginal stenosis occurs, or there are other anatomic issues [3]. It is important to recognize that the obstructed hemiuterus can have normal reproductive function following vaginal septum resection as evidenced by the observation that 23–37 % of pregnancies occur in the side ipsilateral to the vaginal obstruction [4, 19]. Given that the hemiuterus on the obstructed side is reproductively competent, there is little reason to remove it unnecessarily.

Drainage of Hematocolpos

Another option to treat double uterus with obstructed hemivagina is to drain and decompress the hematocolpos. This procedure will immediately relieve the pain due to a dilated hemivagina and uterus. However, drainage must be considered a temporary solution as the obstruction is still there, so with subsequent menstruation the hematocolpos will reaccumulate and the patient will need to undergo another procedure in the future to relieve the obstruction. Drainage and decompression is accomplished by transvaginal or laparoscopic approach, although transvaginal drainage may be associated development of infection and pyocolpos given the bacterial flora in the vagina and perineum [6, 12, 18] (Fig. 12.8). If decompression is performed, then menstruation must be suppressed with combined hormonal contraceptives (oral contraceptives pills), progestins (depo-medroxyprogesterone acetate or norethindrone), or GnRH analogs with add back therapy. If menses are not suppressed, then the hematocolpos will reaccumulate relatively quickly (Fig. 12.9). Another concern with this approach is once the hematocolpos is decompressed, the hematocolpos is smaller and more difficult to locate for subsequent vaginal septum excision and marsupialization. Usually, the patient has to be taken off hormonal suppression and allow one or more menstrual cycles to distend the obstructed vaginal cavity and facilitate septum excision. In these cases, intraoperative ultrasound or placement of a probe through the hemiuterus on the obstructed side and through the cervix to tent the vaginal septum may facilitate localization and resection. Primary resection of vaginal septum is the preferred approach to treat double uterus with obstructed hemivagina. However, drainage and decompression may be utilized when there is uncertainty regarding the exact anatomic configuration, lack of surgical expertise to treat the condition, or other health or social conditions that would make primary resection problematic.

Hormonal suppression of menstruation without first decompressing the hematocolpos is only appropriate if the patient is not in severe pain. It may take several weeks for the hematocolpos to decrease in size in response to the medications. As a result, the patient will continue to have symptoms she presented with for a long time requiring continued pain medication and in some cases hospital admission for pain control.

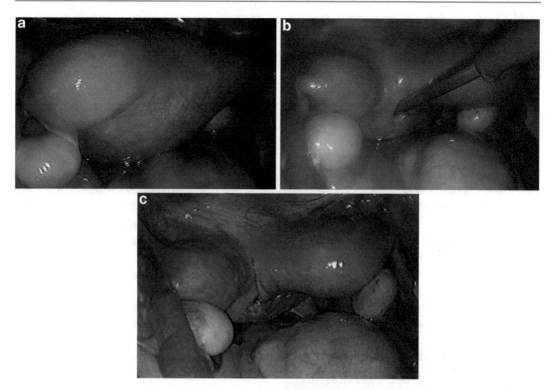

Fig. 12.8 (**a**) Laparoscopic picture showing uterus didelphys with obstructed right hemivagina. The large mass is the hematocolpos. The left uterine horn is visible and not dilated. (**b**) Laparoscopic image showing laparoscopic drainage of the hematocolpos. (**c**) Laparoscopic image showing the decompressed right hematocolpos. The uterus didelphys is easily identified

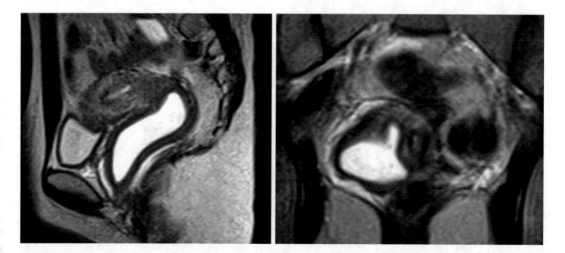

Fig. 12.9 MRI showing reaccumulation of hematocolpos and hematometra 2 months after laparoscopic decompression of right hematocolposin the absence of menstrual suppression

Treatment of Double Uterus and Obstructed Hemivagina with Microperforation

Managing patients who have double uterus and obstructed hemivagina with a microperforation can be challenging as it can be difficult to identify the microperforation. The microperforation may be located in the vaginal septum or there may be a communication between the obstructed and non-obstructed side anywhere along the cervical or uterine septum in the case of complete septate configuration, or between the two cervices or uterine cavities with other anomalies [2, 10, 11] (Fig. 12.10). If the microperforation is located in the vaginal septum, then identifying the perforation may be easier at the time of men-

struation when menstrual blood may be seen at the perforation site. Alternatively, under anesthesia, pressure on the obstructed side will reveal egress of fluid through the microperforation either directly or with the use of vaginoscopy. Once the microperforation is identified, it can be dilated using lacrimal duct probes or a thin tipped clamp such as right angle to gently dilate the opening and identify the vaginal septal tissue. Resection of the vaginal septum then can proceed as usual. If the communication between the two sides is located between the cervices or uterine cavities, then hysterosalpingogram (under anesthesia for an adolescent) can be utilized to identify the location [37] (Fig. 12.11). In these cases, once the vaginal septum is resected on the obstructed side, there is no need to further resect or clarify the communication between the two sides as both sides will drain vaginally.

Impact on Fertility

A few studies have evaluated reproductive function in women who have a history of double uterus with obstructed hemivagina. Due to the inherent delay in diagnosis seen with this disorder and subsequent retrograde menstruation, these individuals are at risk of developing adhesions, hematosalpinx, ovarian endometrioma, and undergoing salpingectomy and ovarian cystectomy or oophorectomy, all of which can adversely affect reproductive function. Interestingly, there does not seem to be an

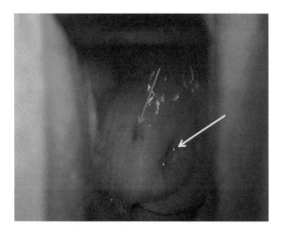

Fig. 12.10 Vaginal view showing normal left cervical os and small lesion representing microperforation in the obstructed right hemivagina

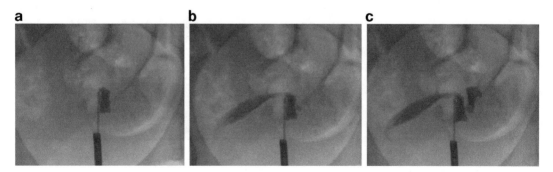

Fig. 12.11 HSG used to identify a communication between the two cervices of a uterus didelphys with obstructed left hemivagina. Catheter placed into the right cervix. (**a**) Radiopaque dye entering the right cervix. (**b**) Radiopaque dye fills the right uterine cavity. Careful eval-

uation reveals a small extravasation of dye coming from the left side of the cervix representing the communication between the two cervices. (**c**) Radiopaque dye filling left cervix from the right side, confirming communication increased rate of primary infertility in these patients with studies reporting conception rates of 62–87 % [4, 19, 21]. Some studies have estimated the rate of spontaneous abortion to be as high as 40 %, most likely related to the uterine anomaly [38]. In the largest series to evaluate reproductive outcome following treatment of double uterus obstructed hemivagina, 33 women attempted conception with 28 women (84.8 %) reporting 52 pregnancies [4]. In another large series of 36 patients, 13 out of 15 patients who wanted children succeeded in conceiving (87 %) with a live birth rate of 77 % [21]. In another retrospective study, 13 out of 21 women (62 %) who attempted pregnancy conceived 22 pregnancies with a live birth rate of 91 % [19]. A smaller retrospective study reported 9 women with 20 pregnancies after septum resection with a live birth rate of 65 % [27]. Pregnancy occurred more commonly in the non-obstructive side, which may reflect prior damage to the ipsilateral tube, ovary, or adhesive disease due to retrograde menstruation with obstruction [4, 19]. However, a significant number of pregnancies have been reported to occur in the uterus ipsilateral to the obstruction with 23 % [19] and 36.5 % [4] reported in the two studies, respectively.

Conclusions

Obstructive Müllerian duct anomalies should be suspected in any adolescent with abdominal pain or cyclic dysmenorrhea, and obstructed hemivagina, HWW syndrome, and OHVIRA syndrome should be included in the differential diagnosis. If left undiagnosed or untreated, an obstructed hemivagina can lead to endometriosis, pelvic adhesions, pyometra, pyosalpinx, or intraabdominal abscesses. Thus, early diagnosis and septum resection should be undertaken to relieve hemivaginal obstruction and circumvent subsequent complications.

References

1. Purslow CE. A case of unilateral haematocolps, haematometria, and haematosalpinx. J Obstet Gynaecol Br Emp. 1922;29:643.
2. Fedele L, Motta F, Frontino G, Restelli E, Bianchi S. Double uterus with obstructed hemivagina and ipsilateral renal agenesis: pelvic anatomic variants in 87 cases. Hum Reprod. 2013;28(6):1580–3.
3. Smith NA, Laufer MR. Obstructed hemivagina and ipsilateral renal anomaly (OHVIRA) syndrome: management and follow-up. Fertil Steril. 2007; 87(4):918–22.
4. Tong J, Zhu L, Lang J. Clinical characteristics of 70 patients with Herlyn-Werner-Wunderlich syndrome. Int J Gynaecol Obstet. 2013;121(2):173–5.
5. Attar R, Yıldırım G, Inan Y, Küzılkale O, Karateke A. Uterus didelphys with an obstructed unilateral vagina and ipsilateral renal agenesis: a rare cause of dysmenorrhoea. J Turk Ger Gynecol Assoc. 2013;14(4):242–5.
6. Schutt AK, Barrett MR, Trotta BM, Stovall DW. Perioperative evaluation in Herlyn-Werner-Wunderlich syndrome. Obstet Gynecol. 2012;120(4):948–51.
7. Heinonen PK. Clinical implications of the didelphic uterus: long-term follow-up of 49 cases. Eur J Obstet Gynecol Reprod Biol. 2000;91:183–90.
8. Cetinkaya SE, Kahraman K, Sonmezer M, Atabekoglu C. Hysteroscopic management of vaginal septum in a virginal patient with uterus didelphys and obstructed hemivagina. Fertil Steril. 2011;96(1):e16–8.
9. Herlyn U, Werner H. Simultaneous occurrence of an open Gartner-duct cyst, a homolateral aplasia of the kidney and a double uterus as a typical syndrome of abnormalities. Geburtshilfe Frauenheilkd. 1971;31:340–7.
10. Del Vescovo R, Battisti S, Di Paola V, Piccolo CL, Cazzato RL, Sansoni I, Grasso RF, Zobel BB. Herlyn-Werner-Wunderlich syndrome: MRI findings, radiological guide (two cases and literature review), and differential diagnosis. BMC Med Imaging. 2012;12:4.
11. Vercellini P, Daguati R, Somigliana E, Viganò P, Lanzani A, Fedele L. Asymmetric lateral distribution of obstructed hemivagina and renal agenesis in women with uterus didelphys: institutional case series and a systematic literature review. Fertil Steril. 2007;87(4):719–24.
12. Gholoum S, Puligandla PS, Hui T, Su W, Quiros E, Laberge JM. Management and outcome of patients with combined vaginal septum, bifid uterus, and ipsilateral renal agenesis (Herlyn-Werner-Wunderlich syndrome). J Pediatr Surg. 2006;41(5):987–92.
13. Grimbizis GF, Campo R. Congenital malformations of the female genital tract: the need for a new classification system. Fertil Steril. 2010;94(2):401–7.
14. Acien P, Acien MI. The history of female genital tract malformation classifications and proposal of an updated system. Hum Reprod Update. 2011; 17(5):693–705.
15. Oppelt P, Renner SP, Brucker S, Strissel PL, Strick R, Oppelt PG, et al. The VCUAM (Vagina Cervix Uterus Adnex-associated Malformation) classification: a new classification for genital malformations. Fertil Steril. 2005;85(5):1493–7.

16. American Fertility Society. The AFS classification of adnexal adhesions, distal tubal occlusion, tubal occlusion secondary to tubal ligation, tubal pregnancies, Mullerian anomalies and intrauterine adhesions. Fertil Steril. 1988;49:944–55.

17. Berger-Chen S, Ritch JM, Kim JH, Evanko J, Hensle TW. An unusual presentation of uterine didelphys and obstructed hemivagina. J Pediatr Adolesc Gynecol. 2012;25(6):e129–31.

18. Khong TL, Siddiqui J, Mallinson P, Horton D, Gandhi J, Daniel R. Herlyn-Werner-Wunderlich syndrome: uterus didelphys, obstructed hemivagina, and ipsilateral renal agenesis-role of sonographically guided minimally invasive vaginal surgery. Eur J Pediatr Surg. 2012;22(2):171–3.

19. Heinonen PK. Pregnancies in women with uterine malformation, treated obstruction of hemivagina and ipsilateral renal agenesis. Arch Gynecol Obstet. 2013;287:975–8.

20. Rock JA, Jones Jr HW. The double uterus associated with an obstructed hemivagina and ipsilateral renal agenesis. Am J Obstet Gynecol. 1980;138:339–42.

21. Candiani GB, Fedele L, Candiani M. Double uterus, blind hemivagina, and ipsilateral renal agenesis: 36 cases and long-term follow-up. Obstet Gynecol. 1997;90:26–32.

22. Paulozzi LJ, Lary JM. Laterality patterns in infants with external birth defects. Teratology. 1999; 60:265–71.

23. Fantel AG, Person RE, Burroughs-Gleim C, Shepard TH, Juchau R, Backler B. Asymmetric development of mitochondrial activity in rat embryos as a determinant of the defect patterns induced by exposure to hypoxia, hyperoxia, and redox cyclers in vitro. Teratology. 1991;44:355–62.

24. Fantel AG, Juchau R, Tracy JW, Burroughs CJ, Person RE. Studies of mechanisms of niridazole-elicited embryotoxicity: evidence against a major role for covalent binding. Teratology. 1989;39:63–74.

25. Pereira N, Anderson SH, Verrecchio ES, Brown MA, Glassner MJ. Hemivaginal septum resection in a patient with a rare variant of Herlyn-Werner-Wunderlich syndrome. J Minim Invasive Gynecol. 2014;21(6):1113–7.

26. Wu TH, Wu TT, Ng YY, Ng SC, Su PH, Chen JY, et al. Herlyn-Werner-Wunderlich syndrome consisting of uterine didelphys, obstructed hemivagina and ipsilateral renal agenesis in a newborn. Pediatr Neonatol. 2012;53(1):68–71.

27. Haddad B, Barranger E, Paniel BJ. Blind hemivagina: long-term follow-up and reproductive performance in 42 cases. Hum Reprod. 1999;14(8):1962–4.

28. Olive DL, Henderson DY. Endometriosis and mullerian anomalies. Obstet Gynecol. 1987;69:412–5.

29. Fedele L, Bianchi S, Di Nola G, Franchi D, Candiani GB. Endometriosis and nonobstructive müllerian anomalies. Obstet Gynecol. 1992;79(4):515–7.

30. Rock JA, Zacur HA, Dlugi AM, Jones HW. Pregnancy success following surgical correction of imperforate hymen and complete transverse septum. Obstet Gynecol. 1982;59:448.

31. Kim TE, Lee GH, Choi YM, Jee BC, Ku SY, Suh CS, et al. Hysteroscopic resection of the vaginal septum in uterus didelphys with obstructed hemivagina: a case report. J Korean Med Sci. 2007;22:766–9.

32. Shih CL, Hung YC, Chen CP, Chien SC, Lin WC. Resectoscopic excision of the vaginal septum in a virgin with uterus didelphys and obstructed unilateral vagina. Taiwan J Obstet Gynecol. 2010;49(1):109–11.

33. Nassif J, Al Chami A, Abu Musa A, Nassar AH, Kurdi A, Ghulmiyyah L. Vaginoscopic resection of vaginal septum. Surg Technol Int. 2012;22:173–6.

34. Dorais J, Milroy C, Hammoud A, Chaudhari A, Gurtcheff S, Peterson CM. Conservative treatment of a Herlyn-Werner-Wunderlich müllerian anomaly variant, noncommunicating hemiuterus with Gartner duct pseudocyst. J Minim Invasive Gynecol. 2011; 18(2):262–6.

35. Wang S, Lang JH, Zhu L, Zhou HM. Duplicated uterus and hemivaginal or hemicervical atresia with ipsilateral renal agenesis: an institutional clinical series of 52 cases. Eur J Obstet Gynecol Reprod Biol. 2013;170:507–11.

36. Sanfilippo JS, Wakim NG, Schikler KN, Yussman MA. Endometriosis in association with uterine anomaly. Am J Obstet Gynecol. 1986;154:39–43.

37. Acien P, Acien M, Sanchez-Ferrer M. Complex malformations of the female genital tract. New types and revision of classification. Hum Reprod. 2004;19:2377–84.

38. Propst AM, Hill III JA. Anatomic factors associated with recurrent pregnancy loss. Semin Reprod Med. 2000;18:341–50.

Erratum to: Müllerian Agenesis: Diagnosis, Treatment, and Future Fertility

Jamie Stanhiser and Marjan Attaran

Erratum to:
Chapter 6 in: S.M. Pfeifer (ed.), *Congenital Müllerian Anomalies*,
DOI 10.1007/978-3-319-27231-3_6

The coauthor of Chapter 6 is Jamie Stanhiser and her name was incorrectly spelled as Stanheiser in the original publication. It has been corrected in the chapter and the volume front matter.

The updated online version of this chapter can be found at
https://doi.org/10.1007/978-3-319-27231-3_6

© Springer International Publishing Switzerland 2018
S.M. Pfeifer (ed.), *Congenital Müllerian Anomalies*, DOI 10.1007/978-3-319-27231-3_13

Index

© Springer International Publishing Switzerland 2016
S.M. Pfeifer (ed.), *Congenital Müllerian Anomalies*, DOI 10.1007/978-3-319-27231-3

Printed in the United States
By Bookmasters